Epidemiology and Treatment of Atrial Fibrillation

Edited by Gabriel Cismaru and Keith Andrew Chan

Published in London, United Kingdom

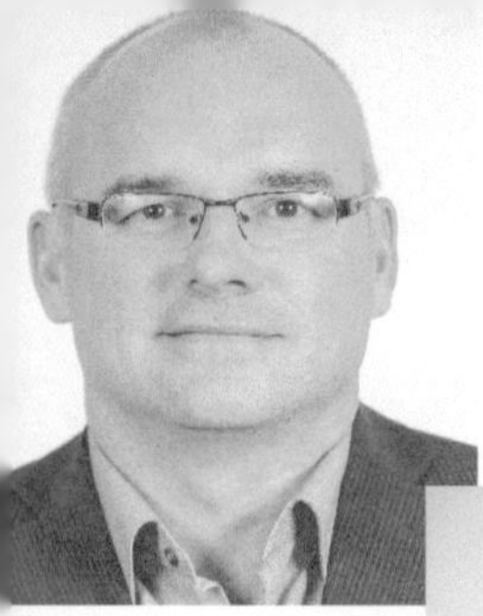
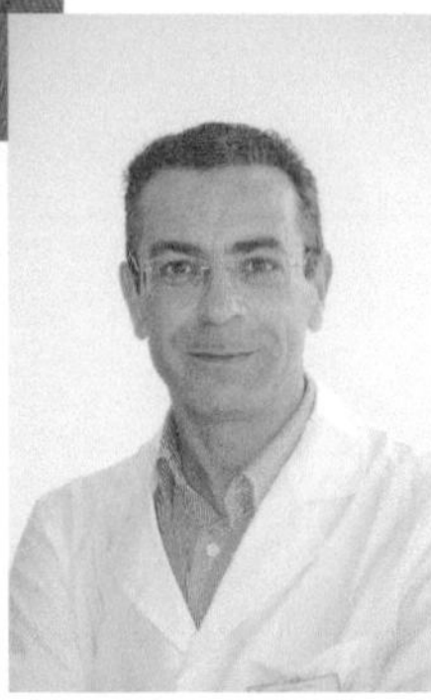
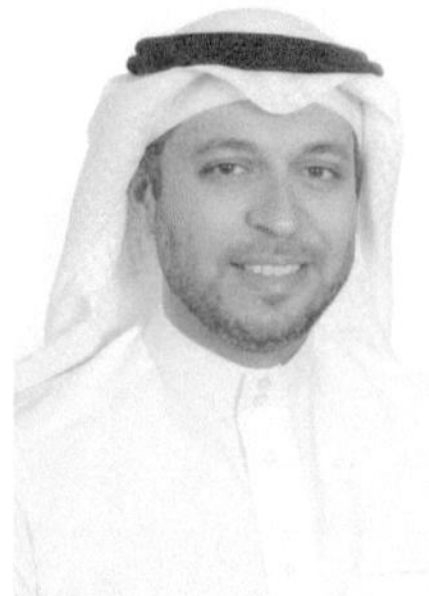
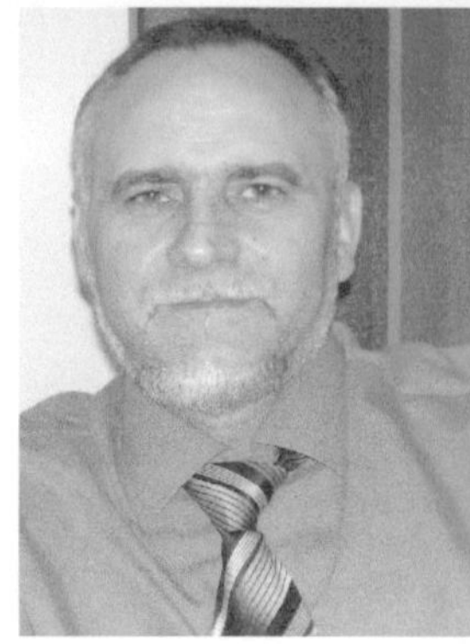
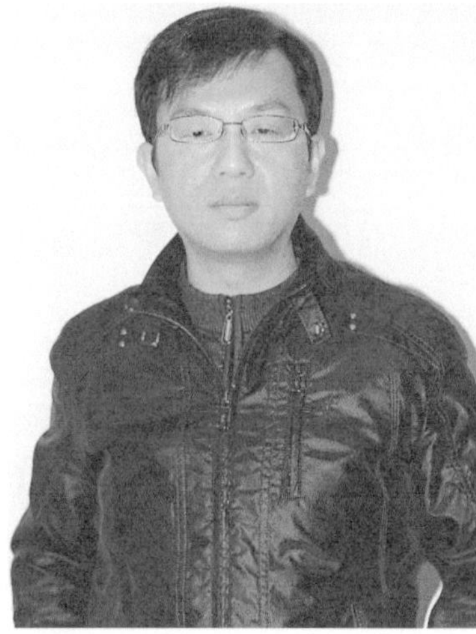
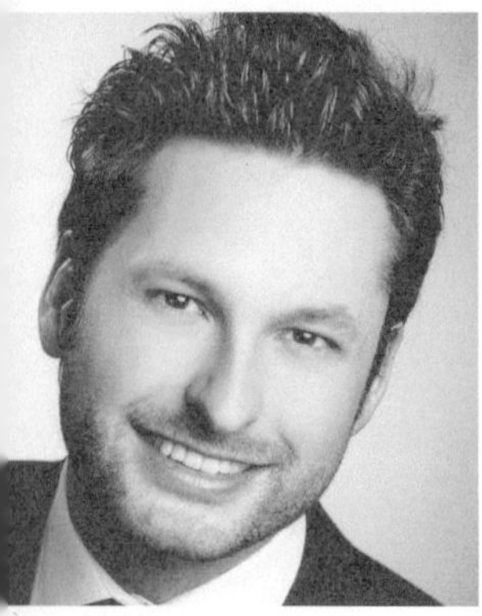
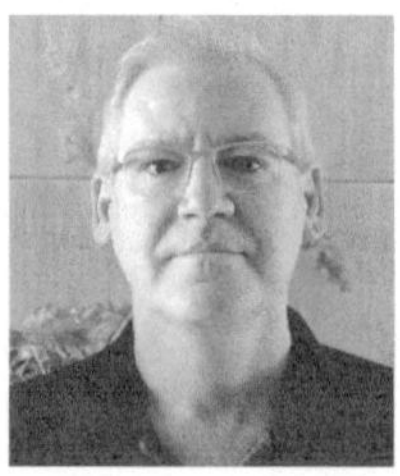

IntechOpen

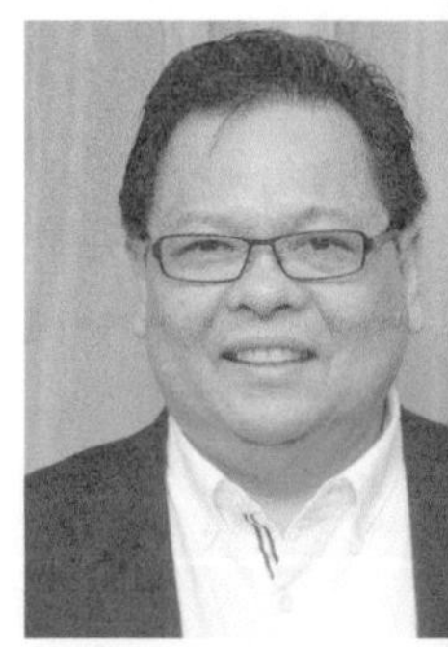
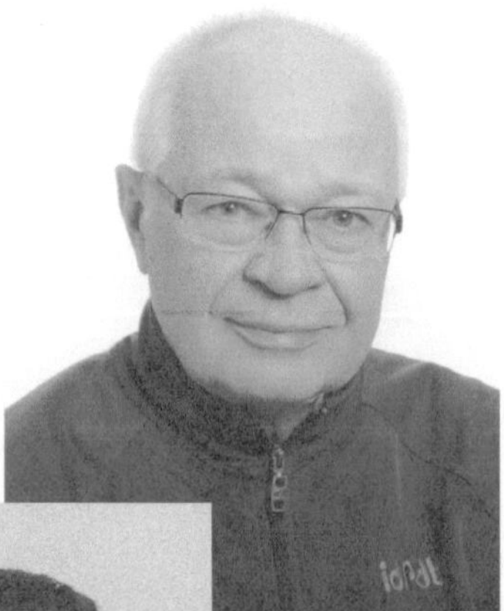
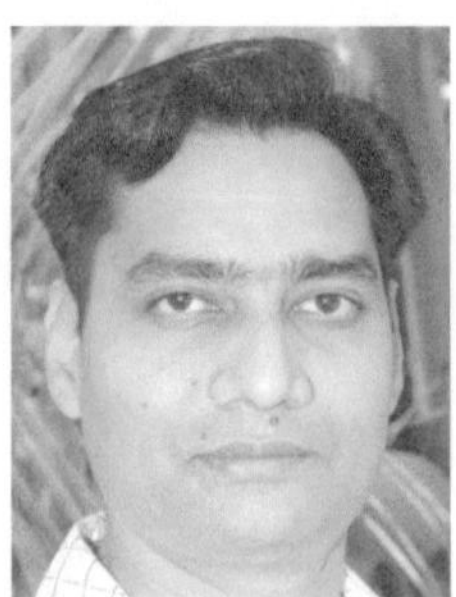
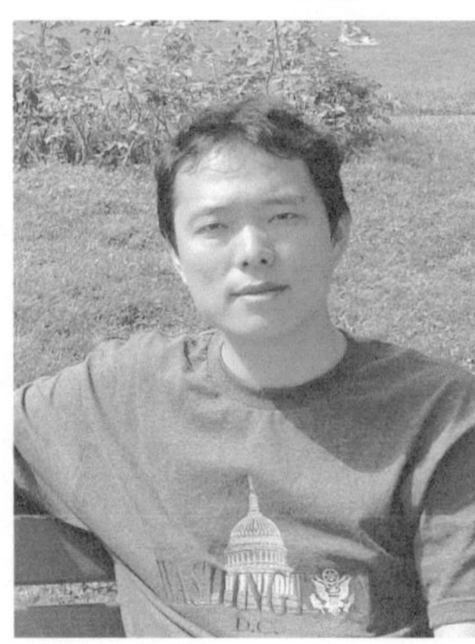
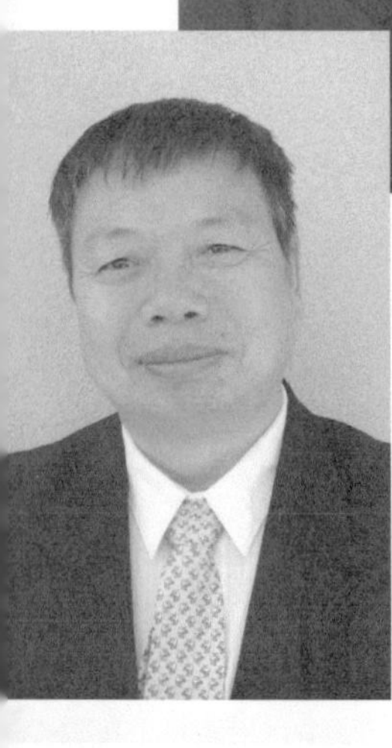
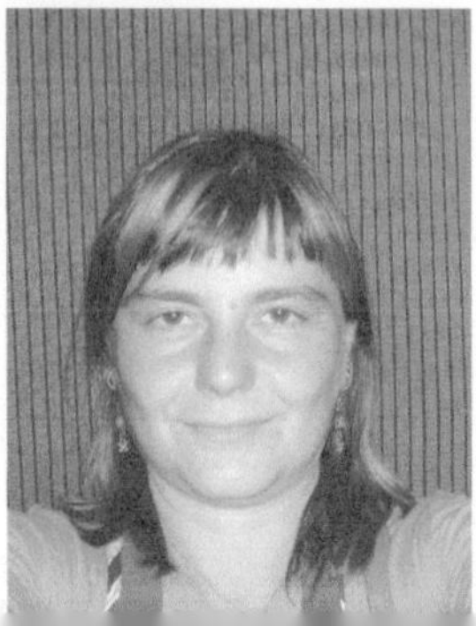

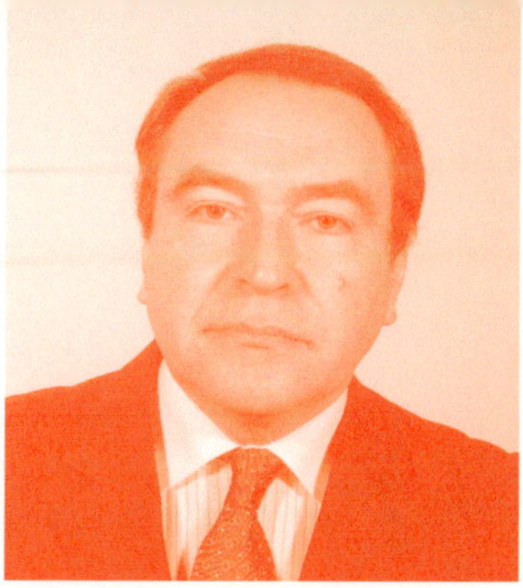
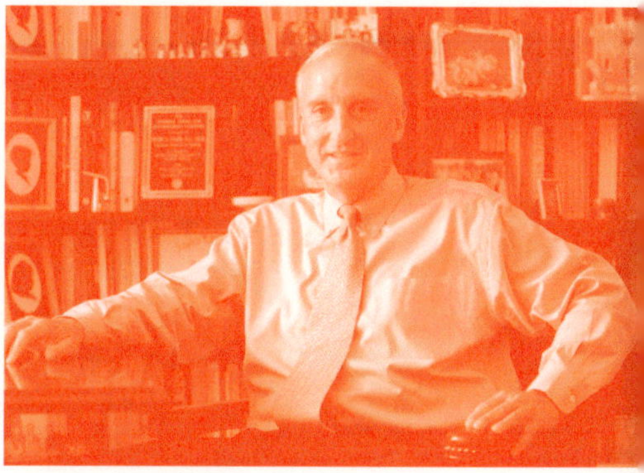
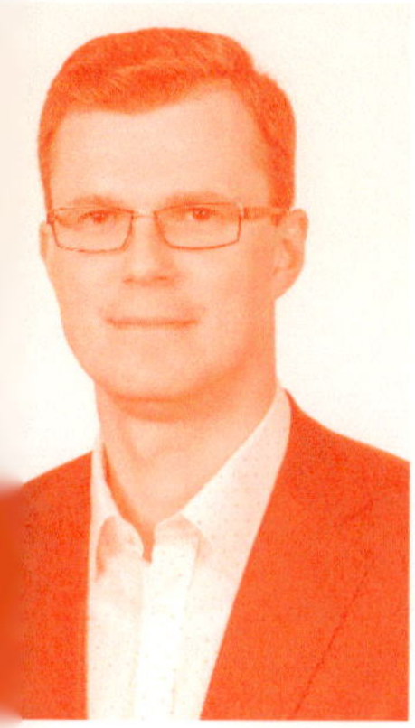
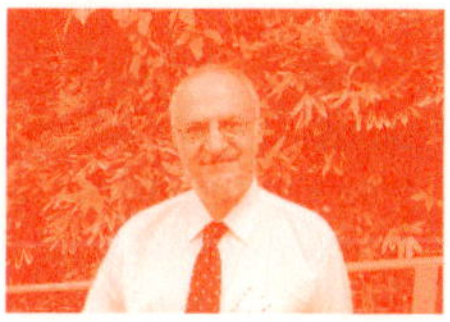
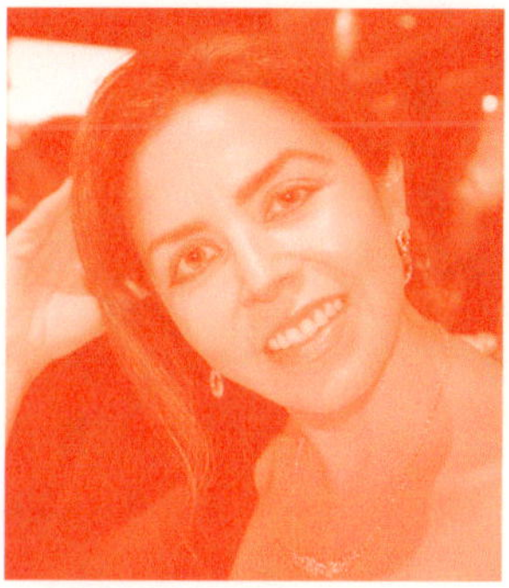

Supporting open minds since 2005

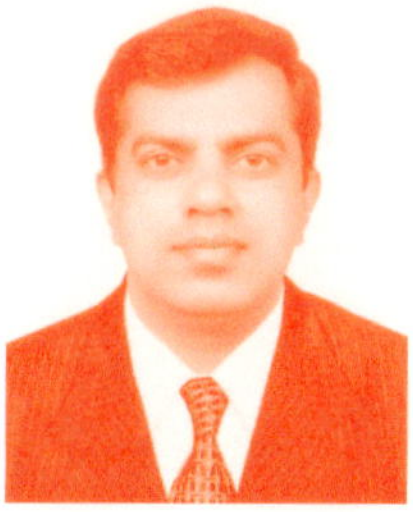
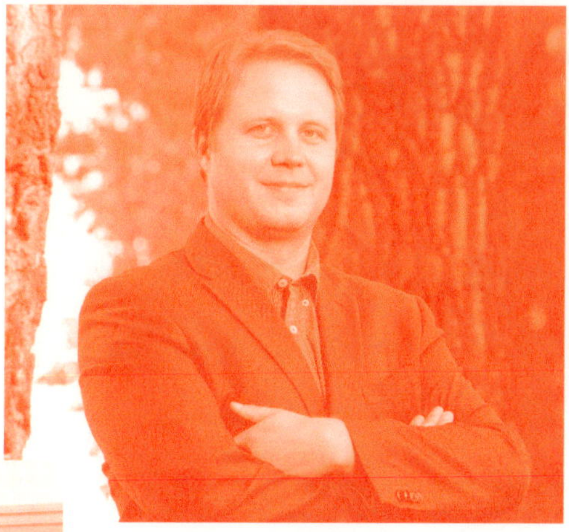
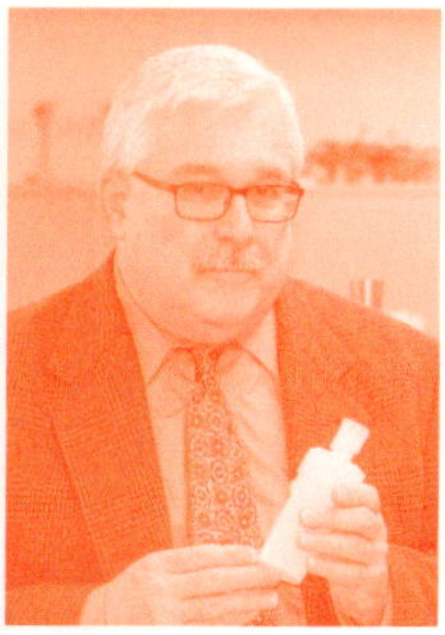
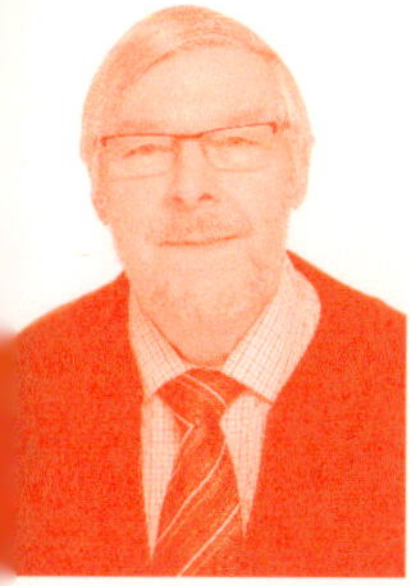
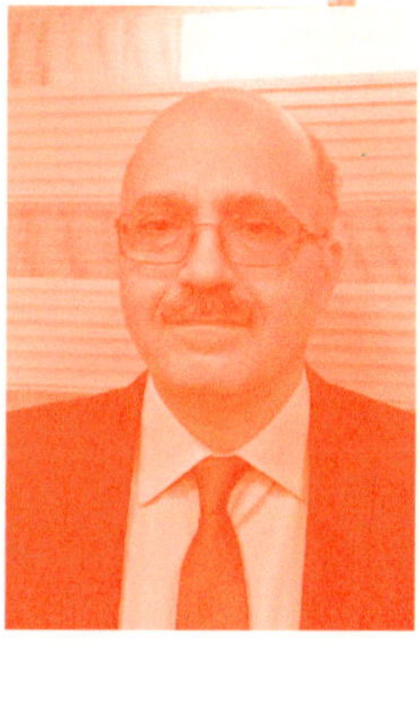
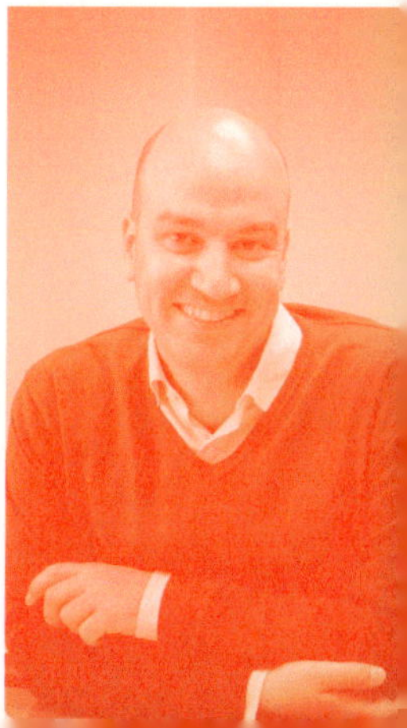
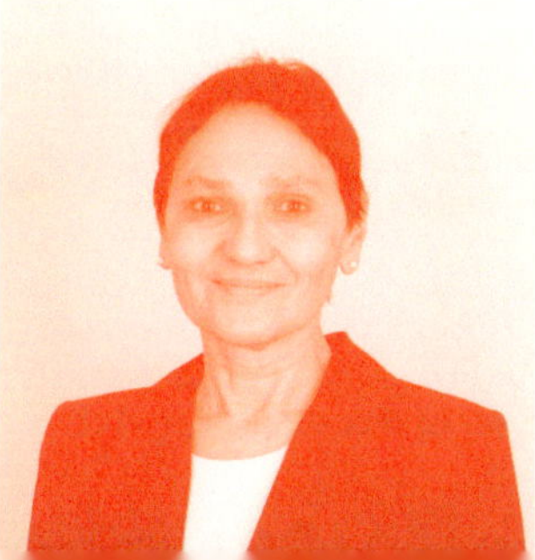

Epidemiology and Treatment of Atrial Fibrillation
http://dx.doi.org/10.5772/intechopen.83059
Edited by Gabriel Cismaru and Keith Andrew Chan

Contributors
Nándor Szegedi, László A Gellér, Andrew Mitchell, Angela Hall, Edward Richardson, Roberto Petidier, Alba Maria Costa, Irene Criado, Stefan Simovic, Ivan Srejovic, Vladimir Zivkovic, Slobodanka Mitrovic, Vladimir Jakovljevic, Jovana Jeremic, Goran Davidovic, Jo Ann LeQuang, Peter Magnusson, Joseph V. Pergolizzi, Randall Wolf, Sunil Ohri, Manoraj Navaratnarajah, Suvitesh Luthra

First published in London, United Kingdom, 2020 by IntechOpen
IntechOpen is the global imprint of INTECHOPEN LIMITED, registered in England and Wales, registration number: 11086078, 7th floor, 10 Lower Thames Street, London, EC3R 6AF, United Kingdom
Printed in Croatia

British Library Cataloguing-in-Publication Data
A catalogue record for this book is available from the British Library

Additional hard and PDF copies can be obtained from orders@intechopen.com

Epidemiology and Treatment of Atrial Fibrillation
Edited by Gabriel Cismaru and Keith Andrew Chan
p. cm.
Print ISBN 978-1-83880-247-9
Online ISBN 978-1-83880-248-6
eBook (PDF) ISBN 978-1-83880-330-8

For EU product safety concerns:
IN TECH d.o.o., Prolaz Marije Krucifikse Kozulić 3, 51000 Rijeka, Croatia, info@intechopen.com or visit our website at intechopen.com.

Meet the editor

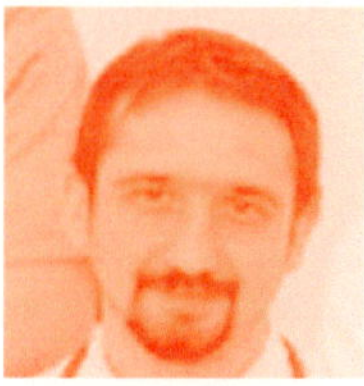

Dr. Gabriel Cismaru is an electrophysiologist who works in the EP lab of the Rehabilitation Hospital Cluj-Napoca. He works in the Cardiac Intensive Care Unit dealing with various cardiac emergencies, including brady- and tachyarrhythmias. A distinguished cardiologist and researcher, Dr. Cismaru has written many articles on catheter ablation of different types of arrhythmias: atrial fibrillation, paroxysmal supraventricular tachycardia, ventricular fibrillation, and a number of books in the field of cardiac arrhythmias.

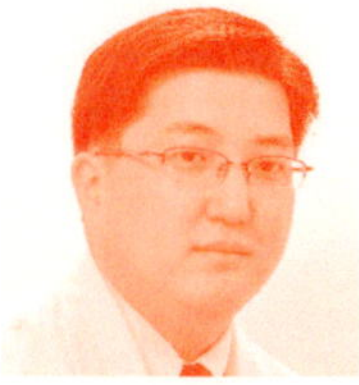

Dr. Keith Andrew Chan graduated from the Cebu Institute of Medicine and pursued his internal medicine residency training at Chong Hua Hospital in Cebu, Philippines. He is currently the Chief Adult Cardiology Fellow of the Chong Hua Heart Institute in Cebu, Philippines. His fields of interest include clinical cardiology, electrophysiology, and arrhythmias as well as interventional and structural cardiology. He is passionate about teaching medical residents and cardiology fellows the basics of hemodynamic and electrophysiologic disease mechanisms and often considers himself a "lifelong student of cardiology."

Contents

Preface

Atrial fibrillation (AF) continues to remain a challenge to both clinical cardiologists and electrophysiology specialists alike. It is the most common type of arrhythmia in Europe and the United States. Advances in the 21st century have brought about new treatment and diagnostic tools that have provided solutions and explanations for numerous problems plaguing early AF management. However, although the optimal management of this highly prevalent arrhythmia has greatly advanced, many challenges are still notable in the wide spectrum of the disease.

Numerous populations encounter atrial fibrillation in their daily lives, with both the elderly and the pediatric population having their own obstacles for optimal management of this arrhythmia. Apart from traditional echocardiographic methods of identifying patients at risk for persistent AF, there are now new methods for traditional cardiac ultrasonography as well as newer modalities that will enable better prognostication and identification of subtypes that will benefit from various AF treatment strategies. Furthermore, with the advent of newer anti-arrhythmic medications and methods of ablation and stroke prevention, the goals of AF treatment have now become easier to achieve—but not without their own share of side effects and adverse events.

The book is divided into two self-contained and distinct parts: the first on the epidemiology of AF and the second on the treatment of this disease. The chapters are well structured, following a logical description, from the epidemiology of the disease, as mentioned before, and continuing with different options of treatment: anticoagulants, antiarrhythmic drugs, catheter ablation, and surgery. The technical information is accompanied by figures or explanatory tables that summarize the information from the text.

Dr. Mitchell Andrew together with his team from Jersey opens the book with a chapter on the prevalence of AF and use of digital technologies to assess the real burden of the disease. Alive Cor, Omron HeartScan, Zio Patch, RhythmPad, InstantChek, and Zenocire EKG are some of the devices used to detect AF, increasing the value of classical methods used for AF detection. These devices will help us see the true face of this widespread arrhythmia in the general population. After the epidemiology of AF is presented, anticoagulation is discussed in the following two chapters: for both the general population and the elderly. Jo Ann LeQuang and her coauthors first define valvular and non-valvular AF using excellent tables that gather information from different European, American, Canadian, Australian, and New Zealand guidelines as well as studies published by experts in the field. After presenting the thromboembolic and bleeding scores, the authors of the chapter describe both antivitamin K and non-antivitamin K anticoagulants. The new oral anticoagulants are presented extensively, using studies on the safety and efficacy of drugs compared to classical antivitamin K. Finally, the authors offer an approach to choose between different anticoagulants based on clinical and lab data. In the following chapter, Petidier Roberto, together with his coauthors from Madrid, Spain, addresses the problems of anticoagulation in a particular category of patients, namely elderly, frail patients. Polymedicines, interactions of different drugs with oral anticoagulants, cognitive and nutritional status, low mobilization due to osteoarticular diseases, swallowing and other digestive problems, cancer, renal failure, and the history of bleeding are delineated by the authors as they are the problems of the third age. All these issues make anticoagulant treatment in the elderly a real challenge, which must be resolved patiently to prevent bleeding or thromboembolic events.

In the fourth chapter, on antiarrhythmic therapy, Simovic Stefan and his coauthors from Serbia describe two approaches for AF: rhythm control and rate control. They then outline each class of antiarrhythmic drug, starting with class I: flecainide and propafenone, class II: betablockers, class III: sotalol, dofetilide, amiodarone, and dronedarone; and ending with new classes of antiarrhythmic drugs, namely vernakalant. The authors also show in a table doses of the drugs, indications, side effects, and mechanisms of action.

In the fifth chapter, Szegedi Nándor with his coauthors from Budapest, Hungary, present the catheter ablation technique for the cure of AF. They start with pulmonary vein isolation for paroxysmal AF, and the techniques that are used today: cryoablation and radiofrequency application with the latest technology available—ablation catheters with pressure sensors and the ablation index to avoid overheating and perforation of the left atrial wall. For persistent AF, the authors present the substrate modification approach associated with pulmonary vein isolation.

In the last chapter, Ohri Sunil and his coauthors from Southampton present the surgical treatment of AF. The authors start with a history of the surgical treatment: left atrial isolation, corridor operation, and atrial transection, techniques that had low success rates and were subsequently replaced by MAZE I, MAZE II, MAZE III, and MAZE IV procedures. Furthermore, they describe other energy sources besides the "cut and sew" technique, such as cryoablation and radiofrequency ablation, microwave, laser, and ultrasound. At the end of their chapter they present evidence from the medical literature on the success rate and safety of the surgical procedures as well as studies comparing the surgical approach with the catheter ablation approach.

On behalf of all authors of this book, we hope that this will serve as a guide to the current body of knowledge on the epidemiology, diagnosis, and treatment of this common arrhythmia and, perhaps, in turn inspire young cardiologists to pursue ambitious careers in electrophysiology.

Dr. Gabriel Cismaru
EP lab of the Rehabilitation Hospital Cluj-Napoca,
Romania

Dr. Keith Andrew Chan
Chief Adult Cardiology Fellow,
Chong Hua Hospital,
Cebu City, Philippines

Section 1

Epidemiology of Atrial Fibrillation

Chapter 1

Screening for Atrial Fibrillation and the Role of Digital Health Technologies

Edward Richardson, Angela Hall and Andrew R.J. Mitchell

Abstract

Atrial fibrillation is the commonest clinical arrhythmia and a leading cause of hospital admission, morbidity and mortality. New digital health technologies are now allowing patients and the general population to identify heart rhythm abnormalities before any encounter with a medical professional. This chapter will include an overview of the prevalence of atrial fibrillation and explore the current recommendations on methods for arrhythmia screening. We discuss different risk factors as well as physiological and structural markers for atrial fibrillation onset. We explore in detail the application of novel digital health technologies such as wearables, watches and mobile devices which may have an impact on screening detection rates. The article concludes with a discussion about how to manage patients with screen detected atrial fibrillation.

Keywords: atrial fibrillation, screening, digital health, wearables, arrhythmia, technology, cardiology, ECG, apple watch, Alivecor, Kardia, Omron HeartScan, Zenicor ECG, Miniscope, Reka e100, Zio Patch, guidelines, Holter monitor, ambulatory ECG, patient centred care, artificial intelligence, iPhone, android, apple, stroke, photoplethysmography

1. Introduction

Atrial fibrillation (AF) is increasing in prevalence with a lifetime risk of one in four people developing this common arrhythmia [1]. Its detection is of rising importance as it is a leading cause of mortality and morbidity. A recent meta-analysis showed a person with AF had an increased risk of all-cause mortality by 46%, of ischaemic heart disease by 61%, of chronic kidney disease by 64%, a 96% higher risk of a major cardiovascular event, and an 88% higher risk of sudden cardiac death. Furthermore, it more than doubled the risk of stroke and increased the risk of congestive heart failure fivefold [2]. Whilst the mechanism behind some of these are unknown, the identification of AF can be used to help reduce the risk of several of the complications, by starting anticoagulation for example. Often persons with AF can be asymptomatic and therefore it may be detected late, such as after a stroke. Around 10% of all ischaemic strokes are associated with a new diagnosis of AF and it is present in around a quarter of all patients with stroke. Screening for AF has received significant focus with a dedicated collaboration established in 2016 called AF Screen. Their aim it is to promote discussion and research about unknown or untreated AF, as a means to reduce stroke and associated mortality [3, 4].

2. Screening

Screening for AF has received considerable attention due to the increasing numbers of patients with the arrhythmia and projections for further increases over the coming years [5]. A variety of screening methods exist from a manual pulse check to the use of novel digital screening tools [3, 6].

Public health screening has increased dramatically over the last few decades through a need and desire to address the growing burden of disease [7]. This exponential growth has been partly achievable through innovations in digital technology and an enhanced ability to detect a growing number of conditions. The rationale for screening is straightforward: detecting disease in its infancy and treating to reduce morbidity, mortality and associated healthcare and societal costs [8]. A paradigm shift has resulted in a more proactive approach whereby early detection of disease has renewed importance over the confines of diagnosis of clinically overt disease. Putting this into context, up to two-thirds of people with AF report that it disrupts their lives [9]. Medical attention may be sought early on, but it is not uncommon for the symptoms of AF to go unnoticed until there is decompensation. If AF is of the paroxysmal nature, it may go undetected unless the practitioner has the insight to investigate symptoms suggestive of an arrhythmia. However, AF can be silent, in other words exhibit no symptoms even in the persistent form and the first diagnosis may not be until there are signs of haemodynamic compromise. Unfortunately it is not uncommon for AF to also be detected when the patient presents with a thromboembolic complication such as stroke [3, 4, 10, 11].

The World Health Organisation lists criteria that should be considered when implementing screening of disease (**Table 1**) [12]. The criteria states that the condition should be an important health problem with accepted treatment. While this work is nearly 50 years old, little has changed in screening criteria. More recent updates suggest consideration of economic implications, quality assurance and informed choice alongside equity and access of screening to the entire target population [7]. This is an important consideration and one yet to achieve consensus in terms of AF screening [13].

Screening approaches vary and include opportunistic, and systematic that can be broken down to targeted, population and mass screening. There remains a lack of consensus regarding the optimal method with a range of studies exploring and evaluating AF screening, with some studies choosing opportunistic, some

1. The condition should be an important health problem.
2. There should be a treatment for the condition.
3. Facilities for diagnosis and treatment should be available.
4. There should be a latent stage of the disease.
5. There should be a test or examination for the condition.
6. The test should be acceptable to the population.
7. The natural history of the disease should be adequately understood.
8. There should be an agreed policy on whom to treat.
9. The total cost of finding a case should be economically balanced in relation to medical expenditure.
10. Case-finding should be a continuous process, not just a "once and for all" project.

Table 1.
Principles and practice of screening for disease [12].

systematic, and others both. In all studies, older age groups are frequently targeted due to perceived cost effectiveness and anticipated positive findings. However, targeting the younger population may help address contributory lifestyle factors, reducing complications that may result. In addition to age, high risk patient groups are further targets for screening. Hypertension, diabetes and heart failure are commonly cited as chronic disease populations at higher risk of cardiovascular complications [11, 14]. As such, these patient groups have often been selected in targeted screening programmes [15–19].

Whilst the European Society of Cardiology guidelines do recommend screening asymptomatic patients for AF, the NICE and the UK National Screening Committee guidance does not [10, 20, 21]. The rationale is the lack of evidence to support it benefiting those identified by screening. This recommendation is currently under review. There are increasing numbers of studies that suggest benefit in screening. A paper in 2014 using the data from the 2004 SAFE trial, showed that of the 78–83% of those identified in the screening for AF were eligible for anticoagulation [22, 23]. Whilst there have been further papers on the cost-effectiveness of screening in AF, unfortunately several of these have continued to rely on the data from the SAFE trial [24]. An ongoing major issue is that few studies have been able to prove better health outcomes from those asymptomatic adults that were screened [25, 26]. This is at least partially due to the difficulty in proving an intervention has prevented a stroke. As such and on the recommendations of collaborations such as AF-SCREEN and the European Society of Cardiology several charities now conduct some level of screening, with most suggesting a simple pulse check [4, 27].

3. Wearable technologies

Digital health technologies have revolutionised health screening, not least within cardiology [28]. Traditional ambulatory Holter monitors (HM) connected by electrodes to the precordium, are still used regularly but have limitations. They can be used for varying lengths of time but can be inconvenient and require laborious analysis. The time and duration of wear may also be incongruent with symptoms and therefore ineffectual [29]. Modern applications can now be utilised through technological advancements, which can enable more ad-hoc monitoring. These vary from new devices to applications on mobile phones. These options can offer more advanced screening with enhanced specificity and sensitivity [29–32].

There are increasing numbers of new technologies being developed that can be used in the screening of AF. We will discuss some of the more well-known options however there will be a focus on the devices where there are published studies that demonstrate their efficacy and diagnostic accuracy. Unfortunately, there are few studies that compare results across the different devices, however, where there is sufficient evidence then we shall try and compare the technologies.

The majority of devices use a single lead, normally analogous to lead I. They do this by providing two electrodes to capture electrical signals from the fingers, thumb, wrist, or palm of each hand [33]. One of the best known is the AliveCor. It has been used in clinical practice since 2011 and there is a plethora of research where AliveCor, or Kardia as it has been more recently branded, has been the tool of choice. The AliveCor has demonstrated high sensitivity and specificity in screening studies and is U.S. Food and Drug Association (FDA) as well as Conformité Européenne (CE) approved [16, 31, 32, 34, 35]. This device creates a single lead, by providing two electrodes for 2 or more fingers of each hand. The data generated is wirelessly transmitted to a smart phone and produces a tracing. The application will notify the user if the tracing is normal or AF. The information can be securely sent to an encrypted AliveCor cloud server or a healthcare professional. The presence of an enhanced filter provides a much smoother tracing. Studies also suggest that even elderly patients found the device easy to use and that it did not restrict activities or cause anxiety [16, 33, 36]. It has been shown to be more likely to diagnose a symptomatic underlying rhythm than an HM [37]. Limiting factors include requiring access to a smartphone and not being recommended for use in children, or those with implanted electronic devices [33, 36].

The Omron HeartScan is another single lead device, similar to the AliveCor. However, with the HeartScan one of the electrodes on the device can also be placed on the chest. It is a stand-alone device so does not require a smart phone, but it is more expensive. There is evidence to suggest that like the AliveCor, it is more likely to successfully diagnose AF, especially if symptomatic, than an HM [33, 38–40].

There are some single lead devices such as the Zio Patch, which aim to provide more continuous monitoring. The Zio Patch is a single use water-resistant adhesive patch similar to a traditional HM but with a few advantages. It can record for longer, 14 days versus 7, and it has no wires, which means it is more discreet and reduces the interference. It is generally well tolerated and studies suggest it may have a higher diagnostic yield for arrhythmia [28, 33, 41–45].

Some other single lead devices are targeted more towards screening. One example, the RhythmPad^{GP}, is designed around the screening of non-symptomatic individuals in a general practice (GP) Surgery. As yet there are no studies showing its efficacy [46]. Another device that is aimed at screening is the Microlife Modified Blood Pressure (BP) monitor. It screens for AF via the detection of an irregularly irregular pulse during the inflation of an automatic blood pressure cuff. BP checks are commonly performed in the primary care setting and increasingly by people in their own homes; the design of the device monopolises on this. The evidence suggests it may even be more accurate than a pulse check [19, 47].

AF detecting devices are ever increasing in number and too numerous to detail here, however, some more well-known examples include: MyDiagnostick, the Reka e100, Miniscope M3, InstantCheck, AfibAlert, and Zenicore EKG. There are less studies associated with these but all show merit in their own way [33, 48–52].

Photoplethysmographic (PPG) technology has also shown promise and works in the same way as a pulse oximeter. Whilst PPG can be more susceptible to movement artefact, [53] they are low cost and widely available commercially including in the Apple Watch and Fitbit [54–56]. Movement artefact can be reduced with the intelligent use of accelerometers in the device [53]. The Cardiio Rhythm smartphone application uses the phone's camera to detect heart rate. It has been shown to be comparable to the AliveCor in sensitivity and specificity [34, 57].

The Apple Watch initially used PPG, however the latest iteration, the Apple Watch 4, now has the ability to perform a single lead ECG. The mechanism is similar to the other single lead ECG devices. One electrode is incorporated in the back of the watch and the second in the crown at the side. The user puts one finger on the crown and is able to obtain an estimation of lead I [56, 58, 59]. Apple are currently funding a study, called the Apple Heart Study, that aims to demonstrate the ability of the Apple Watch to detect previously unknown AF by identifying pulse variability and irregularity. This has the potential to be one of the largest studies on AF identification, with over 400,000 participants, and therefore should be highly powered. Conversely, previous studies are relatively small in size. Additionally, the Apple Heart Study should help provide data for a much wider population than previous studies and therefore potentially help appraise the practicalities of screening large groups [56]. The study has released some preliminary results, which have indicated the Apple watches over all generations had a 71% positive predictive value. The data released also showed that 84% of the time during an irregular pulse notification the patient was in AF [60].

The Apple Heart Study, alongside the GARMIN AF study [61] are part of many ongoing projects; a search of clinical trials revealed frequent utilisation of modern devices within ongoing research projects. The Clinical Trials database exposed 92 trials on a recent search, where screening for AF was the primary outcome [62]. These incorporated an array of screening tools and whilst the majority focused on targeted populations, this was not exclusive. Similarly, the European Union Trials Register revealed 80 studies of a comparable nature, highlighting the ongoing interest in screening for undiagnosed AF [63].

4. Current guidelines

There are multiple different guidelines on the management of AF, in this section we have summarised the areas relating to screening as well as recommendations for anticoagulation.

4.1 European guidelines

The European Society of Cardiology (ESC) 2016 guidelines and recommendations [10] are summarised below with regards to AF screening and stroke prevention in AF:

1. Screening for AF is recommended:

    a. In elderly populations with a suggested age cut off at 65 years on an opportunistic basis.

    b. ECG screening in a more systematic manner may be considered in those at high risk of stroke or aged over 75 years of age.

    c. In Patients with a Transient Ischaemic Attack (TIA) or ischaemic stroke with a short-term ECG recording followed by ECG monitoring for at least 72 hours. There is also the suggestion that non-invasive monitors or implanted loop recorders can also be considered especially in those patients with cryptogenic stroke.

    d. Via Implantable Cardioverter Defibrillators (ICDs) and pacemakers. These should be interrogated on a regular basis for evidence of atrial high rate episodes (AHRE). This is because AHRE are associated with an increased risk of overt AF.

2. Stroke prevention in AF recommendations are:

    a. CHA_2DS_2-VASc Score (**Table 2**) and if the score is equal to or greater than 1 for a male or 2 for a female then oral anticoagulation can be considered. It should also be noted that female sex will only add to the score if another risk factor is present. Anticoagulation should also be continued even if the patient has surgical exclusion or occlusion of their left atrial appendage in at-risk patient groups.

    b. Oral anticoagulation is recommended in the form of a Novel Oral Anticoagulant (NOAC) unless the patient has a mechanical heart valve or moderate to severe mitral stenosis where a vitamin K antagonist (VKA) is recommended. NOACs should also be avoided in women planning a

Risk factor	Points
Congestive heart failure—signs or symptoms of or objective evidence of reduced LVEF	+1
Hypertension—on BP medication or resting BP >140/90 on a minimum of at least two occasions	+1
Age greater than or equal to 75 years old	+2
Diabetes mellitus—on hypoglycaemic agent or fasting glucose of >7 mmol/l (>125 mg/dl)	+1
Previous thromboembolism, including stroke and transient ischaemic attack	+2
Vascular disease—including peripheral artery disease, aortic plaque, or previous myocardial infarction	+1
Age between 65 and 74 years old	+1
Female sex	+1

Table 2.
CHA_2DS_2-VASc modified from ESC guidelines [10].

pregnancy or those that are already pregnant. If a VKA is used then the target International Normalised Ratio (INR) is 2.0–3.0, unless it is required to be higher for another comorbidity. Those on VKAs should have their INRs closely monitored, with the aim to keep the time in the therapeutic range as high as possible. There is also no requirement for genetic testing before the initiation of VKAs as these have been evaluated to have little or no effect on the bleeding risk.

c. Antiplatelet monotherapy is not recommended for the prevention of stroke in patients with AF irrespective of stroke risk. Combinations of antiplatelets and oral anticoagulants should be avoided unless there is another indication for antiplatelet therapy. This is due to the increased risk of bleeding.

d. In patients with stroke and AF immediate anticoagulation with low molecular weight heparin or heparin is not recommended

e. Patients with hypertrophic cardiomyopathy (HCM) that develop AF should have lifelong oral anticoagulation for stroke prevention.

f. Atrial flutter should be treated with ablation of the cavotricuspid isthmus if antiarrhythmic treatment fails, or as a potential first line treatment depending on patient preference. Anticoagulation should be treated under the same guidelines as AF.

g. Oral anticoagulation should be interrupted in patients with severe ongoing, active bleeding, until resolution of the underlying cause.

h. Bleeding risk scores should be considered before starting anticoagulation but with the aim of identifying modifiable risk factors than to recommend the holding of anticoagulants.

4.2 Comparison with American guidelines

The American Heart Association (AHA), American College of Cardiology (ACC), and Heart Rhythm Society (HRS) Guidelines [64] as of their 2019 update

[65, 66] are similar to the ESC guideline. In fact, the major changes in the 2019 compared to the 2014 guideline bring it closer to the ESC guidance. For example, the inclusion of Edoxaban as a NOAC.

More relevantly, the AHA/ACC/HRS guideline moved from referring to "nonvalvular AF" as the exclusion criteria for the CHA_2DS_2-VASc Score to using the narrower criteria of moderate to severe mitral stenosis or a mechanical heart valve. It is also the exclusion criteria for NOACs, as VKA should be used in these patients. This more closely aligns with the ESC guideline. The AHA/ACC/HRS guideline has also changed the classification for women within the CHA_2DS_2-VASc Score; female sex now confers no points if it is the lone risk factor. Both have the same scoring cut-offs for anticoagulation, they also both recommend NOACs over VKAs, in those eligible and similarly do not recommend aspirin in those with low CHA_2DS_2-VASc Score.

However, whilst the ESC guidance does recommend some opportunistic screening as a class I recommendation with level B evidence, the AHA/ACC/HRS guidelines are less forthcoming. Though the American guidance does suggest monitoring in those with cryptogenic stroke including the use of implantable cardiac monitors, such as loop recorders, it does not comment on more generalised screening. Both guidelines recommend interrogating the recordings of those with ICDs or pacemakers for the presence of AHREs, prompting further investigation for AF. The ESC guidance takes this further and acknowledges the recent studies demonstrating the possibilities for a more generalised approach and even recognises the potential role for the new devices mentioned above [10, 51, 64–66].

4.3 Screening after stroke

AF Screening after an ischaemic stroke or TIA is commented on in the ESC guidelines where it recognises how commonly AF is detected in stroke survivors. As mentioned above, not only does it recommend monitoring patients for at least 72 hours it also states that extensive screening should be considered. It is worth noting that the guidelines go as far as to recommend implantable loop recorders in those with "cryptogenic stroke", where no other cause could be identified, such as carotid artery stenosis. This is a class IIa recommendation with Level B evidence.

4.4 Guidance on atrial high rate episodes

AHREs are mentioned in both sets of guidelines. The definition of AHREs can differ but most studies have used a length of greater than 5 minutes as a cut off but some going for a cut off of 6 minutes [67]. The actual atrial rate chosen also varies with some citing 175 bpm and others up to 220 bpm [68–70]. The ESC guideline defines them as lasting 5–6 minutes or greater and a rate faster than 180 bpm [10]. Recent studies have suggested they are quite common with a 30–70% incidence in those with an implantable device [70, 71]. Whilst it is difficult to adjust for confounding factors, AHREs are associated with an elevated risk of stroke, death, and subsequent AF [67]. However, a study in 2017 showed that a temporal relationship between a stroke and an episode of AHRE was only seen in 15% of those with an implanted device [71].

Both the ESC and the AHA/ACC/HRS guidelines recommend further investigation of those patients identified to have AHRE. The AHA/ACC/HRS guideline mainly recommends further investigation to establish if true AF is present [10, 65]. The ESC guideline echoes this, however, suggests the inclusion of patient preference and accepts that rarely anticoagulation may be considered in patients without documented AF.

5. Patient centred care and the role of technology

Both the ESC and NICE recommend that patients be involved in the decision making where possible, as do the AHA/ACC/HRS guidelines to a lesser extent [10, 21, 64–66]. This can be achieved by simply informing them of the risks and benefits of different options, and ideally tailoring them to the patient but advancements in technology means that we may have other ways of individualising care.

Given the AF detecting technologies above, several papers have suggested this may be used to enable patients to self-diagnose and manage their own conditions to a greater or lesser degree depending on the estimated accuracy of the product [53, 56, 72]. This could coalesce perfectly with certain AF treatment strategies such as "pill in the pocket" cardioversion. Other ways this could be useful is in judging the effectiveness of rate or rhythm control in asymptomatic patients [33, 73]. In symptomatic individuals it may also help guide them on when to seek help [33]. Some tracings may even be able to check for complications from medications, such as QT interval monitoring on patients receiving anti-arrhythmic drug therapy [74]. The technology and software in devices such as the Zio patch or Apple watch could allow rate and rhythm monitoring over a longer period of time than would normally be possible without a device such as a loop recorder [38, 41, 48].

Furthermore certain devices, such as the AliveCor, HeartScan, or Apple watch, could be used to capture an ad-hoc single lead ECG for intermittent symptoms [53]. Considering palpitations are a common complaint in primary care and the time limitations on HMs, these devices could enable patients to obtain a reading for symptoms that may be longer than a week apart [16, 39, 73, 75]. They have also been shown to be effective in the paediatric setting [52].

Devices can also be used to provide lifestyle advice, motivation, and educational messages. These can be linked to a daily ECG tracing such as in the ongoing iHEART trial [76]. If this concept were to be expanded, personalised health promotion advice could be provided to patients. This could be extended to providing patients with reminders to take medication and therefore increase their compliance [10, 77]. It could also provide data to patients and researchers alike to establish what, if anything, seem to trigger their symptoms, fast ventricular response, or re-initiation of an episode of AF. Devices could also make it easier to target select groups and enrol them in further research [78, 79]. Additionally, this could provide insights into the demographics of AF and help further narrow down any screening attempts.

While the evidence remains unclear, the level of burden of AF could help dictate the need for anticoagulation in patients. Data gathered at a population and individual level could help personalise the requirement for anticoagulation and the risks thereof [26, 80].

The ESC guidelines recommend the use of technology to support care of patients with AF for multiple reasons. It increases coherent exchange of information between the patient and health care professionals. The guidelines also suggest that it may increase the implementation of evidence-based care, and therefore improve outcomes, by using adjuncts such as decision support software. This may help personalise care for each patient, whilst strengthening adherence to guidelines.

Artificial intelligence (AI) may help personalise care further. AI has been suggested for the diagnosis of AF since the early 1990s [81]. There has even been suggestion more recently that it can be used to predict when AF will occur up to an hour before the event in those with non-permanent AF [82, 83]. AI has many more potential benefits, from helping gather the most useful data on a patient before a consultation to outpatient monitoring and subsequent prioritisation [36, 84–87].

Patients appear to be embracing these new technologies. For example, a recent survey by the Kings Fund [88] showed the majority of people surveyed were willing to use video consultations with their GP especially for minor ailments. The wearables market is also continuing to increase in size, with International Data Corporation's 2017 prediction that the number of wearables sold will almost double by 2021 [89, 90].

There is also an increasing body of evidence that patients having access to their clinical notes and data increases satisfaction and compliance [91, 92]. There is an appetite for patient-controlled records and data. The development of applications such as Apple Health on patients' devices has helped enable patients to keep track of everything from their own BP readings to their list of medications and allergies. Some of these are even more advanced, including GenieMD, which integrate with telemedicine consultations, check for drug interactions, and remind patients when to file for a repeat prescription [93]. Patient controlled records would empower patients and would enable them to take the relevant information with them wherever they go [94–96]. This is not a new concept, it has been used in paper form within maternity [97] and paediatrics [98] settings for a substantial period of time. Evidence shows they are effectively used [99]. Furthermore, there is a move to digitalise both of these [98, 100].

6. Review of the evidence for screening

There are two main types of screening mentioned in the studies, opportunistic and systematic. The evidence shows that an equivocal number of patients were identified with either method [22, 23, 26]. This implies that opportunistic screening is more cost effective [101]. Pulse palpation is an example of this kind of screening and is the limit recommended by the NICE guidance and even then it is under certain indications [21]. Unfortunately pulse palpation lacks specificity [102] and could therefore generate multiple false positives. The novel devices may help improve this as they have been shown to have a better specificity with most being above or around 90% and the lowest being 87%, [26] compared to 71% [101] for pulse palpation alone. Devices can either simulate lead I, use PPG, or BP cuff pulse detection. They have a good sensitivity and specificity, are generally quite easy to use, and therefore may increase the accuracy and feasibility. Whilst they may require further validation with larger studies [33] and more heterogenous populations, some larger studies have still shown them to be cost effective and effective in potential screening scenarios.

The type of screening matters, with targeted and opportunistic screening potentially cost-effective or even cost reducing when aimed at higher risk populations. However, there is limited evidence with regards to the AF detected by these devices having any effect on clinical outcomes, as these were extrapolated from existing studies [6, 16, 32, 34, 103–111]. There is no evidence behind anticoagulation of potentially very short lived runs of AF or AHREs that can be picked up by some devices. Potential harms have not been studied in great depth, nor the cost of incidental findings in these studies [25, 26]. Despite this some of these risks can be mitigated, many devices only simulate one lead or even just pulse pattern, and therefore reduce the chance of picking up other ECG findings, such as T-wave inversion, that may then warrant further investigation.

Given the association between stroke and TIA with AF it is sensible and recommended to include screening in the work up of these patients. Current guidelines suggest the use of ILRs and external loop recorders in those with cryptogenic stroke. The novel devices that provide long term monitoring, rather than short tracings, could be highly useful in these instances. They are less cumbersome and less invasive. The Zio Patch was reported to detect a higher number of arrhythmias than a traditional HM in one study, however, the longer monitoring period may account for this [4, 10, 26, 29, 41, 73, 111].

Those patients identified by screening may need to go on and have further ECGs depending on the method of identification. If the method did not utilise an ECG lead, then the patient will need to have a confirmatory ECG. Once AF is confirmed then rate control or anticoagulation would need to be considered via the CHA_2DS_2-VASc Score in accordance to the guidelines. In some instances, rhythm control may also be considered on an elective basis [10, 64, 65].

7. Conclusion

AF is an important, common disease, with an increasing incidence and the potential for multiple complications. It remains underdiagnosed and could potentially fit the criteria for screening, but the guidelines are divided as to whether this is recommended or not. There are multiple different novel devices that are designed to detect for AF, of which several are beginning to acquire a meaningful evidence base. Such devices might be used to increase the ease and specificity of screening for AF compared to traditional methods, they may also increase the sensitivity. There are multiple clinical trials ongoing where screening for AF is the primary outcome, which should help provide further evidence. However, there still needs to be further research before screening wide populations becomes viable. Further studies are needed comparing the different devices to each other, especially in a screening capacity. There needs to be further research into what duration of AHREs or AF increases the risk of stroke, as well as whether screening really does improve clinical outcomes.

Conflict of interest

The authors confirm that there are no conflicts of interest.

Author details

Edward Richardson, Angela Hall and Andrew R.J. Mitchell*
Department of Cardiology, Jersey General Hospital, St Helier, Jersey

*Address all correspondence to: mail@jerseycardiologist.com

References

[1] Lloyd-Jones DM, Wang TJ, Leip EP, Larson MG, Levy D, Vasan RS, et al. Lifetime risk for development of atrial fibrillation: The Framingham heart study. Circulation. 2004;**110**(9):1042-1046

[2] Odutayo A, Wong CX, Hsiao AJ, Hopewell S, Altman DG, Emdin CA. Atrial fibrillation and risks of cardiovascular disease, renal disease, and death: Systematic review and meta-analysis. BMJ. 2016;**354**:i4482

[3] Engdahl J, Andersson L, Mirskaya M, Rosenqvist M. Stepwise screening of atrial fibrillation in a 75-year-old population: Implications for stroke prevention. Circulation. 2013;**127**(8):930-937

[4] Freedman B, Camm J, Calkins H, Healey JS, Rosenqvist M, Wang J, et al. Screening for atrial fibrillation: A report of the AF-SCREEN international collaboration. Circulation. 2017;**135**(19):1851-1867

[5] Schnabel RB, Yin X, Gona P, Larson MG, Beiser AS, McManus DD, et al. 50 year trends in atrial fibrillation prevalence, incidence, risk factors, and mortality in the Framingham heart study: A cohort study. The Lancet. 2015;**386**(9989):154-162

[6] Jacobs MS, Kaasenbrood F, Postma MJ, van Hulst M, Tieleman RG. Cost-effectiveness of screening for atrial fibrillation in primary care with a handheld, single-lead electrocardiogram device in the Netherlands. EP Europace. 2016;**20**(1):12-18

[7] Andermann A, Blancquaert I, Beauchamp S, Dery V. Revisiting Wilson and Jungner in the genomic age: A review of screening criteria over the past 40 years. Bulletin of the World Health Organization. 2008;**86**(4):317-319

[8] Saquib N, Saquib J, Ioannidis JP. Does screening for disease save lives in asymptomatic adults? Systematic review of meta-analyses and randomized trials. International Journal of Epidemiology. 2015;**44**(1):264-277

[9] Markides V, Schilling RJ. Atrial fibrillation: Classification, pathophysiology, mechanisms and drug treatment. Heart (British Cardiac Society). 2003;**89**(8):939-943

[10] Kirchhof P, Benussi S, Kotecha D, Ahlsson A, Atar D, Casadei B, et al. 2016 ESC guidelines for the management of atrial fibrillation developed in collaboration with EACTS. Europace: European Pacing, Arrhythmias, and Cardiac Electrophysiology: Journal of the Working Groups on Cardiac Pacing, Arrhythmias, and Cardiac Cellular Electrophysiology of the European Society of Cardiology. 2016;**50**(5):e1-e88

[11] Krishnamoorthy S, Lip GY. Hypertension, stroke and the impact of atrial fibrillation. Expert Review of Cardiovascular Therapy. 2008;**6**(10):1287-1289

[12] Wilson JM, Glover JG, Organization WH. Principles and practice of screening for disease. The Journal of the Royal College of General Practitioners. 1968;**16**(4):318

[13] Lown M, Moran P. Should we screen for atrial fibrillation? BMJ. 2019;**364**:l43

[14] Kotecha D, Piccini JP. Atrial fibrillation in heart failure: What should we do? European Heart Journal. 2015;**36**(46):3250-3257

[15] Davis RC, Hobbs FD, Kenkre JE, Roalfe AK, Iles R, Lip GY, et al. Prevalence of atrial fibrillation in the general population and in high-risk groups: The ECHOES study. Europace:

European Pacing, Arrhythmias, and Cardiac Electrophysiology: Journal of the Working Groups on Cardiac Pacing, Arrhythmias, and Cardiac Cellular Electrophysiology of the European Society of Cardiology. 2012;**14**(11): 1553-1559

[16] Halcox JPJ, Wareham K, Cardew A, Gilmore M, Barry JP, Phillips C, et al. Assessment of remote heart rhythm sampling using the AliveCor heart monitor to screen for atrial fibrillation: The REHEARSE-AF study. Circulation. 2017;**136**(19):1784-1794

[17] Samol A, Masin M, Gellner R, Otte B, Pavenstadt HJ, Ringelstein EB, et al. Prevalence of unknown atrial fibrillation in patients with risk factors. Europace: European Pacing, Arrhythmias, and Cardiac Electrophysiology: Journal of the Working Groups on Cardiac Pacing, Arrhythmias, and Cardiac Cellular Electrophysiology of the European Society of Cardiology. 2013;**15**(5): 657-662

[18] Verberk WJ, Omboni S, Kollias A, Stergiou GS. Screening for atrial fibrillation with automated blood pressure measurement: Research evidence and practice recommendations. International Journal of Cardiology. 2016;**203**:465-473

[19] Wiesel J, Arbesfeld B, Schechter D. Comparison of the microlife blood pressure monitor with the Omron blood pressure monitor for detecting atrial fibrillation. The American Journal of Cardiology. 2014;**114**(7): 1046-1048

[20] King S, Fitzgerald A, Bartlett C, Mahon J, Arber M, Carr E, et al. Evidence Summary for Screening for Atrial Fibrillation in Adults. External Review against Programme Appraisal Criteria for the UK National Screening Committee. London: UK National Screening Committee; 2018

[21] National Clinical Guideline C. National Institute for Health and Clinical Excellence: Guidance. Atrial Fibrillation: The Management of Atrial Fibrillation. London: National Institute for Health and Care Excellence (UK); 2014

[22] Fitzmaurice DA, Hobbs FD, Jowett S, Mant J, Murray ET, Holder R, et al. Screening versus routine practice in detection of atrial fibrillation in patients aged 65 or over: Cluster randomised controlled trial. BMJ. 2007; **335**(7616):383

[23] Swancutt D, Hobbs R, Fitzmaurice D, Mant J, Murray E, Jowett S, et al. A randomised controlled trial and cost effectiveness study of systematic screening (targeted and total population screening) versus routine practice for the detection of atrial fibrillation in the over 65s: (SAFE) [ISRCTN19633732]. BMC Cardiovascular Disorders. 2004;**4**:12

[24] Welton NJ, McAleenan A, Thom HH, Davies P, Hollingworth W, Higgins JP, et al. Screening strategies for atrial fibrillation: A systematic review and cost-effectiveness analysis. Health Technology Assessment. 2017;**21**(29): 1-236

[25] Jonas DE, Kahwati LC, Yun JDY, Middleton JC, Coker-Schwimmer M, Asher GN. Screening for atrial fibrillation with electrocardiography: Evidence report and systematic review for the US preventive services task force. Journal of the American Medical Association. 2018;**320**(5):485-498

[26] Zungsontiporn N, Link MS. Newer technologies for detection of atrial fibrillation. BMJ. 2018;**363**:k3946

[27] Lobban T, Breakwell N, Hamedi N, Antoniou S, Alves De Costa F, Tous S, et al. Identifying the undiagnosed AF patient through "know your pulse" community pharmacy based events held

in ten countries during arrhythmia Alliance world heart rhythm week 2017. European Heart Journal. 2018;**39** (suppl_1):263

[28] Turakhia MP, Desai SA, Harrington RA. The outlook of digital health for cardiovascular medicine: Challenges but also extraordinary opportunities. JAMA Cardiology. 2016; **1**(7):743-744

[29] Zimetbaum P, Goldman A. Ambulatory arrhythmia monitoring: Choosing the right device. Circulation. 2010;**122**(16):1629-1636

[30] Harris K, Edwards D, Mant J. How can we best detect atrial fibrillation? The Journal of the Royal College of Physicians of Edinburgh. 2012;**42** (Suppl 18):5-22

[31] Lau JK, Lowres N, Neubeck L, Brieger DB, Sy RW, Galloway CD, et al. iPhone ECG application for community screening to detect silent atrial fibrillation: A novel technology to prevent stroke. International Journal of Cardiology. 2013;**165**(1):193-194

[32] Lowres N, Neubeck L, Salkeld G, Krass I, McLachlan AJ, Redfern J, et al. Feasibility and cost-effectiveness of stroke prevention through community screening for atrial fibrillation using iPhone ECG in pharmacies. The SEARCH-AF study. Thrombosis and Haemostasis. 2014;**111**(6):1167-1176

[33] Bansal A, Joshi R. Portable out-of-hospital electrocardiography: A review of current technologies. Journal of Arrhythmia. 2018;**34**(2):129-138

[34] Chan PH, Wong CK, Poh YC, Pun L, Leung WW, Wong YF, et al. Diagnostic performance of a smartphone-based Photoplethysmographic application for atrial fibrillation screening in a primary care setting. Journal of the American Heart Association. 2016;**5**(7):e003428

[35] Chan P-H, Wong C-K, Pun L, Wong Y-F, Wong MM-Y, Chu DW-S, et al. Head-to-head comparison of the AliveCor heart monitor and microlife WatchBP office AFIB for atrial fibrillation screening in a primary care setting. Circulation. 2017;**135**(1):110-112

[36] National Institute for Health and Care Excellence. AliveCor Heart Monitor and AliveECG app (Kardia Mobile) for detecting atrial fibrillation. National Institute for Health and Care Excellence. 2015. Report No.: 978-1-4731-1373-2 [Accessed: 05 June 2019]

[37] Reed MJ, Grubb NR, Lang CC, O'Brien R, Simpson K, Padarenga M, et al. Multi-Centre randomised controlled trial of a smart phone-based event recorder alongside standard care versus standard care for patients presenting to the emergency department with palpitations and pre-syncope - the IPED (investigation of palpitations in the ED) study: Study protocol for a randomised controlled trial. Trials. 2018;**19**(1):711

[38] de Asmundis C, Conte G, Sieira J, Chierchia GB, Rodriguez-Manero M, Di Giovanni G, et al. Comparison of the patient-activated event recording system vs. traditional 24 h Holter electrocardiography in individuals with paroxysmal palpitations or dizziness. Europace: European Pacing, Arrhythmias, and Cardiac Electrophysiology: Journal of the Working Groups on Cardiac Pacing, Arrhythmias, and Cardiac Cellular Electrophysiology of the European Society of Cardiology. 2014;**16**(8): 1231-1235

[39] Kaleschke G, Hoffmann B, Drewitz I, Steinbeck G, Naebauer M, Goette A, et al. Prospective, multicentre validation of a simple, patient-operated electrocardiographic system for the detection of arrhythmias and electrocardiographic changes. Europace: European Pacing, Arrhythmias, and

Cardiac Electrophysiology: Journal of the Working Groups on Cardiac Pacing, Arrhythmias, and Cardiac Cellular Electrophysiology of the European Society of Cardiology. 2009;**11**(10): 1362-1368

[40] Kearley K, Selwood M, Van den Bruel A, Thompson M, Mant D, Hobbs FR, et al. Triage tests for identifying atrial fibrillation in primary care: A diagnostic accuracy study comparing single-lead ECG and modified BP monitors. BMJ Open. 2014; **4**(5):e004565

[41] Barrett PM, Komatireddy R, Haaser S, Topol S, Sheard J, Encinas J, et al. Comparison of 24-hour Holter monitoring with 14-day novel adhesive patch electrocardiographic monitoring. The American Journal of Medicine. 2014;**127**(1):95.e11-95.e17

[42] Rosenberg MA, Samuel M, Thosani A, Zimetbaum PJ. Use of a noninvasive continuous monitoring device in the management of atrial fibrillation: A pilot study. Pacing and Clinical Electrophysiology. 2013;**36**(3): 328-333

[43] Schreiber D, Sattar A, Drigalla D, Higgins S. Ambulatory cardiac monitoring for discharged emergency department patients with possible cardiac arrhythmias. The Western Journal of Emergency Medicine. 2014; **15**(2):194-198

[44] Tung CE, Su D, Turakhia MP, Lansberg MG. Diagnostic yield of extended cardiac patch monitoring in patients with stroke or TIA. Frontiers in Neurology. 2015;**5**:266

[45] Walsh JA 3rd, Topol EJ, Steinhubl SR. Novel wireless devices for cardiac monitoring. Circulation. 2014; **130**(7):573-581

[46] Cardiocity. RhythmPadGP. Available from: http://www.cardiocity.com/?portfolio=rhythm-pad-gp [Accessed: 06 June 2019]

[47] Wiesel J, Fitzig L, Herschman Y, Messineo FC. Detection of atrial fibrillation using a modified microlife blood pressure monitor. American Journal of Hypertension. 2009;**22**(8): 848-852

[48] Doliwa PS, Frykman V, Rosenqvist M. Short-term ECG for out of hospital detection of silent atrial fibrillation episodes. Scandinavian Cardiovascular Journal. 2009;**43**(3): 163-168

[49] Rekhviashvili A, Baganashvili E, Tan K, Raymakers F, Sakandelidze T. Reproducibility and diagnostic value of E100 event recorder for patients with complains on heart arrhythmias and no changes on multiple routine ECGs and 24-hour holter monitoring. Georgian Medical News. 2012;**203**:29-33

[50] Schuchert A, Behrens G, Meinertz T. Evaluation of infrequent episodes of palpitations with a patient-activated hand-held electrocardiograph. Zeitschrift für Kardiologie. 2002;**91**(1): 62-67

[51] Tieleman RG, Plantinga Y, Rinkes D, Bartels GL, Posma JL, Cator R, et al. Validation and clinical use of a novel diagnostic device for screening of atrial fibrillation. Europace: European Pacing, Arrhythmias, and Cardiac Electrophysiology: Journal of the Working Groups on Cardiac Pacing, Arrhythmias, and Cardiac Cellular Electrophysiology of the European Society of Cardiology. 2014;**16**(9): 1291-1295

[52] Usadel L, Haverkämper G, Herrmann S, Löber R, Weiss K, Opgen-Rhein B, et al. Arrhythmia detection in pediatric patients: ECG quality and diagnostic yield of a patient-triggered Einthoven Lead-I event recorder

(Zenicor EKG-2™). Pediatric Cardiology. 2016;**37**(3):491-496

[53] Eerikainen LM, Bonomi AG, Schipper F, Dekker LRC, Vullings R, de Morree HM, et al. Comparison between electrocardiogram- and photoplethysmogram-derived features for atrial fibrillation detection in free-living conditions. Physiological Measurement. 2018;**39**(8): 084001

[54] Allen J. Photoplethysmography and its application in clinical physiological measurement. Physiological Measurement. 2007;**28**(3):R1-R39

[55] Haghayegh S, Khoshnevis S, Smolensky MH, Diller KR. Accuracy of PurePulse photoplethysmography technology of Fitbit charge 2 for assessment of heart rate during sleep. Chronobiology International. 2019; **36**(7):927-933

[56] Turakhia MP, Desai M, Hedlin H, Rajmane A, Talati N, Ferris T, et al. Rationale and design of a large-scale, app-based study to identify cardiac arrhythmias using a smartwatch: The apple heart study. American Heart Journal. 2019;**207**:66-75

[57] Yan BP, Chan CK, Li CK, To OT, Lai WH, Tse G, et al. Resting and postexercise heart rate detection from fingertip and facial photoplethysmography using a smartphone camera: A validation study. JMIR mHealth and uHealth. 2017; **5**(3):e33

[58] Apple. Apple Watch Series—Health. 2019. Available from: https://www.apple.com/apple-watch-series-4/health/ [Accessed: 06 June 2019]

[59] Apple. Taking an ECG with the ECG app on Apple Watch Series 4. 2019. Available from: https://support.apple.com/en-us/HT208955 [Accessed: 06 June 2019]

[60] Stanford University School of Medicine. Apple Heart Study demonstrates ability of wearable technology to detect atrial fibrillation. Available from: http://med.stanford.edu/news/all-news/2019/03/apple-heart-study-demonstrates-ability-of-wearable-technology.html [Accessed: 17 June 2019]

[61] U.S. National Library of Medicine. Atrial Fibrillation Detection Using Garmin Wearable Technology (GARMIN AF). 2018 NCT03566836.

[62] Clinical Trial Database [Internet]. Available from: https://clinicaltrials.gov/ [Accessed: 06 June 2019]

[63] EU Clinical Trials Register [Internet]. Available from: https://www.clinicaltrialsregister.eu/ [Accessed: 06 June 2019]

[64] January CT, Wann LS, Alpert JS, Calkins H, Cigarroa JE, Cleveland JC Jr, et al. 2014 AHA/ACC/HRS guideline for the management of patients with atrial fibrillation: Executive summary: A report of the American College of Cardiology/American Heart Association task force on practice guidelines and the Heart Rhythm Society. Circulation. 2014;**130**(23):2071-2104

[65] January CT, Wann LS, Calkins H, Chen LY, Cigarroa JE, Cleveland JC Jr, et al. 2019 AHA/ACC/HRS focused update of the 2014 AHA/ACC/HRS guideline for the Management of Patients with Atrial Fibrillation: A report of the American College of Cardiology/American Heart Association task force on clinical practice guidelines and the Heart Rhythm Society. Journal of the American College of Cardiology. 2019;**74**(1):104-132

[66] January CT, Wann LS, Calkins H, Field ME, Chen LY, Furie KL, et al. AHA/ACC/HRS focused update of the 2014 AHA/ACC/HRS guideline for the Management of Patients with Atrial

Fibrillation: A report of the American College of Cardiology/American Heart Association task force on clinical practice guidelines and the Heart Rhythm Society. Heart Rhythm. 2019; **64**(21):e1-e76

[67] Camm AJ, Simantirakis E, Goette A, Lip GY, Vardas P, Calvert M, et al. Atrial high-rate episodes and stroke prevention. Europace: European Pacing, Arrhythmias, and Cardiac Electrophysiology: Journal of the Working Groups on Cardiac Pacing, Arrhythmias, and Cardiac Cellular Electrophysiology of the European Society of Cardiology. 2017;**19**(2): 169-179

[68] Glotzer TV, Hellkamp AS, Zimmerman J, Sweeney MO, Yee R, Marinchak R, et al. Atrial high rate episodes detected by pacemaker diagnostics predict death and stroke: Report of the atrial diagnostics ancillary study of the MOde selection trial (MOST). Circulation. 2003;**107**(12): 1614-1619

[69] Kawakami H, Nagai T, Saito M, Inaba S, Seike F, Nishimura K, et al. Clinical significance of atrial high-rate episodes for thromboembolic events in Japanese population. Heart Asia. 2017; **9**(2):e010954

[70] Dhutia H. Impact and Management of Atrial High Rate Events Detected by Implantable Cardiac Devices. British Cardiovascular Society Editorial [Internet]. 2017. Available from: https://www.bcs.com/pages/news_full.asp?NewsID=19792648 [Accessed: 08 June 2019]

[71] Freedman B, Boriani G, Glotzer TV, Healey JS, Kirchhof P, Potpara TS. Management of atrial high-rate episodes detected by cardiac implanted electronic devices. Nature Reviews Cardiology. 2017;**14**(12):701-714

[72] Giron NA, Millan CA, Lopez DM. Systematic review on features extracted from PPG signals for the detection of atrial fibrillation. Studies in Health Technology and Informatics. 2019;**261**: 266-273

[73] Turakhia MP, Hoang DD, Zimetbaum P, Miller JD, Froelicher VF, Kumar UN, et al. Diagnostic utility of a novel leadless arrhythmia monitoring device. The American Journal of Cardiology. 2013;**112**(4):520-524

[74] Garabelli P, Stavrakis S, Albert M, Koomson E, Parwani P, Chohan J, et al. Comparison of QT interval readings in Normal sinus rhythm between a smartphone heart monitor and a 12-Lead ECG for healthy volunteers and inpatients receiving Sotalol or Dofetilide. Journal of Cardiovascular Electrophysiology. 2016;**27**(7):827-832

[75] Abi Khalil C, Haddad F, Al Suwaidi J. Investigating palpitations: The role of Holter monitoring and loop recorders. BMJ. 2017;**358**:j3123

[76] Hickey KT, Hauser NR, Valente LE, Riga TC, Frulla AP, Masterson Creber R, et al. A single-center randomized, controlled trial investigating the efficacy of a mHealth ECG technology intervention to improve the detection of atrial fibrillation: The iHEART study protocol. BMC Cardiovascular Disorders. 2016;**16**:152

[77] Peleg M, Michalowski W, Wilk S, Parimbelli E, Bonaccio S, O'Sullivan D, et al. Ideating Mobile health behavioral support for compliance to therapy for patients with chronic disease: A case study of atrial fibrillation management. Journal of Medical Systems. 2018; **42**(11):234

[78] Baca-Motes K, Edwards AM, Waalen J, Edmonds S, Mehta RR, Ariniello L, et al. Digital recruitment and enrollment in a remote nationwide trial of screening for undiagnosed atrial fibrillation: Lessons from the randomized, controlled mSToPS trial.

Contemporary Clinical Trials Communications. 2019;**14**:100318

[79] Guo X, Vittinghoff E, Olgin JE, Marcus GM, Pletcher MJ. Volunteer participation in the health eHeart study: A comparison with the US population. Scientific Reports. 2017;7(1):1956

[80] Glotzer TV, Ziegler PD. Silent atrial fibrillation as a stroke risk factor and anticoagulation indication. The Canadian Journal of Cardiology. 2013;**29** (7 Suppl):S14-S23

[81] Yang TF, Devine B, Macfarlane PW. Artificial neural networks for the diagnosis of atrial fibrillation. Medical and Biological Engineering and Computing. 1994;**32**(6):615-619

[82] Chesnokov YV. Complexity and spectral analysis of the heart rate variability dynamics for distant prediction of paroxysmal atrial fibrillation with artificial intelligence methods. Artificial Intelligence in Medicine. 2008;**43**(2):151-165

[83] Ebrahimzadeh E, Kalantari M, Joulani M, Shahraki RS, Fayaz F, Ahmadi F. Prediction of paroxysmal atrial fibrillation: A machine learning based approach using combined feature vector and mixture of expert classification on HRV signal. Computer Methods and Programs in Biomedicine. 2018;**165**:53-67

[84] Buch VH, Ahmed I, Maruthappu M. Artificial intelligence in medicine: Current trends and future possibilities. British Journal of General Practice. 2018;**68**(668):143-144

[85] Fernandes CO, Lucena CJ. A software framework for remote patient monitoring by using multi-agent systems support. JMIR Medical Informatics. 2017;**5**(1):e9

[86] Rialle V, Lamy JB, Noury N, Bajolle L. Telemonitoring of patients at home: A software agent approach. Computer Methods and Programs in Biomedicine. 2003;**72**(3):257-268

[87] Shahid N, Rappon T, Berta W. Applications of artificial neural networks in health care organizational decision-making: A scoping review. PLoS One. 2019;**14**(2):e0212356

[88] Castle-Clarke S. What will new technology mean for the NHS and its patients?: The Kings Fund and Nuffield Trust. 2018. Available from: https://www.kingsfund.org.uk/sites/default/files/2018-06/NHS_at_70_what_will_new_technology_mean_for_the_NHS_0.pdf

[89] Lamkin P. Wearable Tech Market To Double By 2021: Forbes. 2017. Available from: https://www.forbes.com/sites/paullamkin/2017/06/22/wearable-tech-market-to-double-by-2021/#619dc577d8f3 [Accessed: 09 June 2019]

[90] Yang H, Yu J, Zo H, Choi M. User acceptance of wearable devices: An extended perspective of perceived value. Telematics and Informatics. 2016;**33**(2):256-269

[91] DesRoches CM, Bell SK, Dong Z, Elmore J, Fernandez L, Fitzgerald P, et al. Patients managing medications and Reading their visit notes: A survey of OpenNotes participants. Annals of Internal Medicine. 2019;**171**(1):69-71

[92] Jacob JA. Patient access to physician notes is gaining momentum. Journal of the American Medical Association. 2016;**315**(23):2510-2511

[93] GenieMD. Available from: https://geniemd.com/ [Accessed: 13 June 2019]

[94] Archer N, Fevrier-Thomas U, Lokker C, McKibbon KA, Straus SE. Personal health records: A scoping review. Journal of the American Medical Informatics Association. 2011;**18**(4):515-522

[95] Dameff C, Clay B, Longhurst CA. Personal health records: More promising in the smartphone era? Journal of the American Medical Association. 2019; **321**(4):339-340

[96] Davies P. Should patients be able to control their own records? BMJ [British Medical Journal]. 2012;**345**:e4905

[97] Hamilton SG. Obstetric record card for use in general practice. The Practitioner. 1956;**176**(1051):79-81

[98] Health Policy Team. Personal Child Health Record (PCHR): Royal College of Paediatrics and Child Health. Available from: https://www.rcpch.ac.uk/resources/personal-child-health-record-pchr [Accessed: 09 June 2019]

[99] Walton S, Bedford H, Dezateux C. Use of personal child health records in the UK: Findings from the millennium cohort study. BMJ. 2006;**332**(7536): 269-270

[100] Hawley G, Jackson C, Hepworth J, Wilkinson SA. Sharing of clinical data in a maternity setting: How do paper hand-held records and electronic health records compare for completeness? BMC Health Services Research. 2014;**14**: 650

[101] Hobbs FD, Fitzmaurice DA, Mant J, Murray E, Jowett S, Bryan S, et al. A randomised controlled trial and cost-effectiveness study of systematic screening (targeted and total population screening) versus routine practice for the detection of atrial fibrillation in people aged 65 and over. The SAFE study. Health Technology Assessment. 2005;**9**(40):iii-iv, ix-x):1-74

[102] Taggar JS, Coleman T, Lewis S, Heneghan C, Jones M. Accuracy of methods for detecting an irregular pulse and suspected atrial fibrillation: A systematic review and meta-analysis. European Journal of Preventive Cardiology. 2016;**23**(12):1330-1338

[103] Berge T, Brynildsen J, Larssen HKN, Onarheim S, Jenssen GR, Ihle-Hansen H, et al. Systematic screening for atrial fibrillation in a 65-year-old population with risk factors for stroke: Data from the Akershus cardiac examination 1950 study. Europace: European Pacing, Arrhythmias, and Cardiac Electrophysiology: Journal of the Working Groups on Cardiac Pacing, Arrhythmias, and Cardiac Cellular Electrophysiology of the European Society of Cardiology. 2018;**20**(Fi_3): f299-f305

[104] Chan N-Y, Choy C-C. Screening for atrial fibrillation in 13 122 Hong Kong citizens with smartphone electrocardiogram. Heart. 2017;**103**(1): 24-31

[105] Chan P-H, Wong C-K, Pun L, Wong Y-F, Wong MM-Y, Chu DW-S, et al. Diagnostic performance of an automatic blood pressure measurement device, microlife WatchBP home a, for atrial fibrillation screening in a real-world primary care setting. BMJ Open. 2017;**7**(6):e013685

[106] Kaasenbrood F, Hollander M, Rutten FH, Gerhards LJ, Hoes AW, Tieleman RG. Yield of screening for atrial fibrillation in primary care with a hand-held, single-lead electrocardiogram device during influenza vaccination. Europace: European Pacing, Arrhythmias, and Cardiac Electrophysiology: Journal of the Working Groups on Cardiac Pacing, Arrhythmias, and Cardiac Cellular Electrophysiology of the European Society of Cardiology. 2016;**18**(10): 1514-1520

[107] Svennberg E, Engdahl J, Al-Khalili F, Friberg L, Frykman V, Rosenqvist M. Mass screening for untreated atrial fibrillation: The STROKESTOP study. Circulation. 2015;**131**(25):2176-2184

[108] Tavernier R, Wolf M, Kataria V, Phlips T, Huys R, Taghji P, et al.

Screening for atrial fibrillation in hospitalised geriatric patients. Heart. 2018;**104**(7):588-593

[109] Turakhia MP, Ullal AJ, Hoang DD, Than CT, Miller JD, Friday KJ, et al. Feasibility of extended ambulatory electrocardiogram monitoring to identify silent atrial fibrillation in high-risk patients: The screening study for undiagnosed atrial fibrillation (STUDY-AF). Clinical Cardiology. 2015;**38**(5): 285-292

[110] Wiesel J, Salomone TJ. Screening for atrial fibrillation in patients≥ 65 years using an automatic blood pressure monitor in a skilled nursing facility. The American Journal of Cardiology. 2017; **120**(8):1322-1324

[111] Aronsson M, Svennberg E, Rosenqvist M, Engdahl J, Al-Khalili F, Friberg L, et al. Cost-effectiveness of mass screening for untreated atrial fibrillation using intermittent ECG recording. Europace: European Pacing, Arrhythmias, and Cardiac Electrophysiology: Journal of the Working Groups on Cardiac Pacing, Arrhythmias, and Cardiac Cellular Electrophysiology of the European Society of Cardiology. 2015;**17**(7): 1023-1029

Section 2

Treatment of Atrial Fibrillation

Chapter 2

Anticoagulation in Atrial Fibrillation Patients

Peter Magnusson, Joseph V. Pergolizzi Jr, Randall K. Wolf, Morten Lamberts and Jo Ann LeQuang

Abstract

Atrial fibrillation (AF) is the most common arrhythmia and may cause thromboembolic events, typically stroke. Advances in pharmacological approaches to anticoagulation and groundbreaking large randomized controlled trials of non-vitamin K antagonist oral anticoagulants (NOACs) have changed the paradigm of anticoagulation therapy. Furthermore, observational studies support the efficacy and safety of NOAC. Few studies address the differences among NOACs, but prescriptions should be based on a thorough understanding of their pharmacological differences, including interactions, side effects, reversibility, and practical approach. In a subset of patients with AF, warfarin may still be the preferable option. Consequently, an individualized approach to oral anticoagulation is crucial.

Keywords: anticoagulation, apixaban, atrial fibrillation, dabigatran, edoxaban, rivaroxaban, vitamin K antagonist, warfarin

1. Introduction: the changing paradigm for anticoagulation

Atrial fibrillation (AF) is a prevalent arrhythmia possessing a well-known association with thromboembolic events, especially stroke. In AF, atrial pumping ends, and blood tends to pool in the left atrium rather than be pumped into the left ventricle. Thrombi can form in the sluggish blood pool in the atrial region known as the left atrial appendage (LAA). A typical LAA thrombus can cause stroke or peripheral embolism should it break free. Indeed, AF-related strokes tend to be more life-threatening than strokes caused by other reasons [1].

Anticoagulation therapy prevents strokes and warfarin; the most commonly used vitamin K antagonist (VKA) has been the standard agent used to reduce stroke risk in certain AF patients with risk factors since the 1950s [2]. Historically, warfarin has been the drug of choice, but it has often been underused due to its narrow risk-benefit interval and the need for frequent monitoring. It is being gradually eclipsed by a variety of non-vitamin-K antagonist oral anticoagulants (NOACs) that are demonstrating excellent safety and effectiveness without the need for frequent monitoring and subsequent dose adjustment.

The availability of several pharmacological approaches to anticoagulation as well as a more thorough understanding of risk factors for embolization and bleeding has improved patient care but also complicated prescribing choices. The paradigm for anticoagulation in AF patients has changed. In addition, there are now options for patients that suffer from AF but who, for one reason or another, are unable to take anticoagulants. These patients can often undergo closure of the LAA, the site of the majority of the thrombi.

2. Valvular vs. nonvalvular atrial fibrillation

The distinction between valvular and nonvalvular AF is not helpful in terms of defining the nature of the arrhythmia, but it may be of value in better defining the patient's risk for thromboembolism and which type of anticoagulation therapy (if any) is indicated [3]. AF may be paroxysmal or persistent, for example, or symptomatic or asymptomatic ("silent"). When decisions concerning anticoagulation are to be reached, the main factors that may affect prescribing choices are valvular versus nonvalvular forms of AF. Moreover, it should be noted that patients with nonvalvular AF may have concomitant valvular heart disease.

2.1 Nonvalvular AF

In 2016, the European Society of Cardiology (ESC) defined nonvalvular AF as an exclusion of moderate to severe mitral valve stenosis or metallic prosthetic heart valves [4]. The American Heart Association (AHA) and American College of Cardiology (ACC) went a bit further in the exclusion and stated nonvalvular AF was AF not associated with rheumatic mitral stenosis, metallic or bioprosthetic heart valves, or mitral valve repair [5]. It has even been stated by experts that perhaps the terms "nonvalvular" and "valvular" AF are outmoded and no longer useful. See **Table 1**.

Anticoagulation therapy helps to mitigate the risk of stroke in patients with nonvalvular forms of AF [14]. As such, anticoagulation may be indicated for patients with nonvalvular AF, but other factors may come into play. Surgery can affect the anticoagulation decision, both in terms of whether the AF patient needs anticoagulation therapy before and after surgery or just perioperatively for a short window of time [6].

2.2 Valvular AF

As seen in **Table 1**, valvular heart disease encompasses such conditions as mitral stenosis, mitral regurgitation, aortic stenosis, and aortic insufficiency. Valvular heart disease has an age-dependent prevalence of about 0.7% for 18–44-year-olds and 13.3% in patients ≥75 years, and it is considered a risk factor for stroke and systemic embolism. Valvular heart disease may coexist with arrhythmias, including AF [15]. Prosthetic heart valves are associated with thrombin growth, and heart valve surgery may expose the blood pool to mechanical hardware, both of which may activate intrinsic coagulation pathways. Valvular AF has been associated with platelet activation, which may contribute to further thromboembolic risk [3]. Since patients with mechanical heart valves were considered to be at risk for thromboembolism, they should always be prescribed with VKA for anticoagulation as no data exist for the use of NOAC in this subgroup [13]. Distinguishing characteristics for valvular and nonvalvular heart diseases appear in **Table 2**.

2.3 Other patient populations

AF is a prevalent condition and occurs in many patient subpopulations that merit a short discussion in terms of anticoagulation and AF classification.

Society or source	Definition of valvular AF	Definition of nonvalvular AF
American College of Cardiology Expert Consensus 2017 [6]	AF associated with rheumatic mitral stenosis, a mechanical or bioprosthetic heart valve, or mitral valve repair	All AF not associated with rheumatic mitral stenosis, a mechanical or bioprosthetic heart valve, or mitral valve repair
American College of Chest Physicians 2018 [7]	Moderate to severe mitral stenosis or mechanical heart valve	AF not associated with moderate to severe mitral stenosis or mechanical heart valve
Canadian Cardiovascular Society 2016 [8]	Rheumatic mitral stenosis, mitral valve repair, mechanical or bioprosthetic heart valve	AF not associated with mitral stenosis, mitral valve repair, and mechanical or bioprosthetic heart valve
Canadian Cardiovascular Society 2018 [9]	Rheumatic mitral stenosis, moderate to severe non-rheumatic mitral stenosis, or mechanical heart valve	AF not associated with rheumatic mitral stenosis, moderate to severe non-rheumatic mitral stenosis, or mechanical heart valve
De Caterina, Camm (Expert Opinion) 2016 [10]	Proposes the use of "mechanical and rheumatic mitral AF" or MARM-AF as alternative	AF not associated with mechanical and rheumatic mitral AF
European Heart Rhythm Association and European Society of Cardiology Working Group on Thrombosis 2017 [11]	The term is outdated and should be replaced by a functional Evaluated Heartvalves, Rheumatic or Artificial (EHRA) category, based on the anticoagulation therapy used. EHRA typically is described as Types 1 and 2 Type 1 is valvular heart disease requiring VKA anticoagulation Type 2 is valvular heart disease requiring VKA or NOAC therapy	
European Society of Cardiology 2016 [4]	Avoids the term, preferring "AF related to hemodynamically significant mitral stenosis or prosthetic mechanical heart valves"	AF not related to hemodynamically significant mitral stenosis or prosthetic mechanical heart valves
National Heart Foundation of Australia/Cardiac Society of Australia and New Zealand 2018 [12]	Moderate to severe mitral stenosis or mechanical heart valve	AF not associated with moderate to severe mitral stenosis or mechanical heart valve
UMBRIA-Fibrillazione Atriale Study (Clinical Trial) 2019 [13]	Favors the term Type 2 valvular heart disease, defined as moderate to severe mitral or aortic regurgitation, moderate to severe aortic stenosis, or mild mitral stenosis (mitral valve areas >2.0 cm^2 on echocardiography)	AF not associated with moderate to severe mitral or aortic regurgitation, moderate to severe aortic stenosis, or mild mitral stenosis

Table 1.
The definitions for nonvalvular and valvular AF, which can be crucial to selecting appropriate anticoagulation therapy, are blurred and may even be outmoded. Note that some guidelines did not define these terms at all.

2.3.1 Transcatheter aortic valve procedures

Transcatheter aortic valve replacement (TAVR) is often recommended for low-risk patients with severe symptomatic aortic stenosis, but less is elucidated about the role of postsurgical anticoagulation therapy in this population [16]. TAVR candidates have a 40% rate of pre-existing AF and a further 10% chance of developing new-onset AF following TAVR [17]. Most patients discharged following TAVR (n = 16,694) are on dual antiplatelet therapy without anticoagulation (81.1%) [18].

Aspects of heart disease	Valvular heart disease Type 1	Valvular heart disease Type 2	Nonvalvular AF	Comments
Aortic regurgitation		Yes		
Aortic stenosis			Yes	High risk for stroke
Mechanical heart valve	Yes			High risk for thromboembolism
Mild mitral stenosis		Yes		
Mitral regurgitation		Yes		Common form of valvular heart disease
Moderate to severe aortic stenosis			Yes	
Moderate to severe mitral stenosis	Yes			May be of rheumatic origin

Table 2.
An overview of distinguishing characteristics for valvular heart disease (Types 1 and 2) versus nonvalvular heart disease [13].

In a study of 172 patients who underwent TAVR plus a pacemaker implant, 25% of the patients developed new-onset AF or atrial flutter over the median follow-up period of 15 months. Of these patients, 14.7% had at least an episode of asymptomatic AF, which was detected by device diagnostics in the pacemaker but not on their electrocardiogram (ECG). The cumulative incidence of stroke in this population was 1.4% for patients in normal sinus rhythm compared to 12.5% for new-onset AF patients. Patients with obvious AF, detected on ECG, were significantly more likely to be given anticoagulation therapy than those with subclinical new-onset AF (70% vs. 15%, respectively, $p = 0.02$) [19]. The rate and characteristics of AF in this particular patient population as well as those with new transcatheter aortic valve implantation (TAVI) are not extensively studied.

2.3.2 Catheter ablation patients

Patients undergoing catheter ablation for AF typically receive perioperative anticoagulation treatment that is discontinued following surgery providing they have no other risk factors. In the Role of Coumadin in Preventing Thromboembolism in AF Patients Undergoing Catheter Ablation (COMPARE) study, it was shown that continuing warfarin for 48 hours after the procedure was associated with fewer periprocedural strokes and fewer minor bleeding events compared to bridging using low-molecular-weight heparin [20].

Results are mixed in terms of the safety and effectiveness of warfarin versus newer agents. In a prospective cohort of 290 AF ablation patients, periprocedural administration of dabigatran compared to warfarin was associated with a higher rate of thromboembolic events (2.1% vs. 0.0% for dabigatran and warfarin, respectively) and major bleeding complications (6% vs. 1%, $p = 0.019$) [21]. However, in a case-control analysis of 763 patients undergoing radio-frequency AF ablation, dabigatran patients had similar anticoagulation effectiveness and safety compared to warfarin patients [22]. A meta-analysis of 14 studies on the use of dabigatran vs. warfarin for periprocedural anticoagulation in patients undergoing catheter ablation for AF ($n = 4782$) reported dabigatran patients had a similar incidence of major bleeding events and thromboembolic events compared to warfarin patients, and both agents were associated overall with low rates of complications [23].

NOACs have been evaluated in patients undergoing catheter ablation for AF. In the RE-CIRCUIT, it was shown that uninterrupted dabigatran is associated with fewer bleeding complications than uninterrupted warfarin in this population [24]. The AXAFA-NET 5 trial found that continuous apixaban is safe and effective following catheter ablation to treat AF in terms of bleeding, stroke, and cognitive function [25]. Uninterrupted rivaroxaban was shown to be feasible in this population with event rates similar to that of uninterrupted VKA [26].

2.3.3 Cardiac implantable electronic device patients

In some cases, patients on anticoagulation therapy are subsequently indicated for implantation of a cardiac implantable electronic device (CIED). In a randomized study of patients undergoing implantation of an implantable cardioverter defibrillator (ICD), 343 patients were randomized either to undergo bridging to heparin during the procedure or to be continued on warfarin. Major thromboembolic complications in this study were rare and similar between groups (the heparin patients reported one case of cardiac tamponade and one case of myocardial infarction, while the warfarin group had one transient ischemic attack). Device pocket hematoma of clinical significance occurred in 3.5% of warfarin patients compared to 16.0% of heparin patients [27].

2.3.4 Clinically silent AF

The prevalence of asymptomatic or "clinically silent" (subclinical) AF is unknown but likely substantial [28]. Clinically silent AF is often captured by device diagnostics in CIED patients. In a study of dual-chamber pacemaker patients (411 without known AF and 267 with known AF), it was found that at a median 38 months of follow-up, 30% of those without known AF had silent AF verifiable by the pacemaker. Risk factors for silent AF in this study were heart failure ($p = 0.03$) and age > 75 years ($p = 0.0002$). Sixty-two percent of patients who developed silent AF ($n = 125$) were administered with anticoagulation therapy; of those with known AF at implant ($n = 216$), 80% took anticoagulation therapy. The annual rate of stroke was 1.9% for patients who developed silent AF postimplant compared to 2.1% for those with known AF at implant. Vascular dementia developed in 11.2% of those with known AF at implant compared to 6.2% of those who developed silent AF postimplant ($p = 0.048$) [29].

2.3.5 Clinically silent stroke

Silent stroke may be defined as asymptomatic cerebral infarction, which is typically discovered when brain lesions are found during imaging procedures. Indeed, silent stroke is one of the most common incidental findings in brain scans [30]. The incidence and prevalence of this condition is not known nor are risk factors, although it appears that patients with AF are at elevated risk compared to those without this arrhythmia [31, 32]. The role of anticoagulation for patients at risk for silent stroke is not clear [30].

3. Risk stratification for thrombosis

The goal of anticoagulation therapy in AF patients is to reduce their risk for stroke or systemic embolism. The CHA_2DS_2-VASc scoring system has been developed to calculate the numerous factors that may increase the likelihood of thrombus: hypertension, heart failure, older age, diabetes, stroke, transient ischemic attack, vascular disease, and female sex [5, 33]. For patients who score ≥ 1 on this scoring metric, oral anticoagulation therapy is preferred over antiplatelet therapy. However, scoring tools are imperfect. A large retrospective review of 140,420 AF patients found the annual rate for ischemic stroke with those scoring ≤1 was lower than previously stated (0.1–0.2% for women and 0.5–0.7% for men) [33]. A retrospective cohort study found that age between 65 and 74 years was a stronger predictor of stroke compared to the other items on the CHA_2DS_2-VASc scoring system. People in that age bracket had an annual stroke risk of 1.78%. By the same token, AF patients <50 years of age had low risk (0.53%) [34].

4. Safety issues and bleeding risks

Hemostatic alteration introduces the risk of potentially devastating bleeding, typically intracranial hemorrhage [35]. The consequences of a bleeding event are of greater clinical importance than the amount of bleeding itself, for instance, a small amount of pericardial bleeding following cardiac surgery may have potentially life-threatening consequences, while a much larger bleeding event may be clinically manageable. Bleeding is a high-risk situation and is not the subject of clinical trials. In fact, most of the evidence about bleeding rates and risks is derived from safety reports in clinical trials. Thus, expert consensus often overrides data-driven evidence in terms of bleeding risks.

In addition to procedure-related bleeding risks, individual patient factors for bleeding must also be taken into account. The HAS-BLED score, based on a survey of almost 4000 patients in the Euro Heart Survey on AF, offers a way to create a numerical score based on several factors. The acronym encapsulates some of the key risks: hypertension, abnormal renal/liver function, stroke, bleeding history or predisposition, labile international normalized ratio, elderly (>65 years), and drugs and/or alcohol concomitantly [36]. The HAS-BLED has seen a wide adoption, but two important points must be considered. Firstly, many risk factors in the HAS-BLED score are shared with other risk-scoring schemes for calculating the risk of thrombosis, e.g., hypertension and stroke. Secondly, a high HAS-BLED score is not necessarily indicative that oral anticoagulation should be omitted but may be used to select patients in need for regular follow-up.

5. Drug therapies and prescribing options

For over half a century, the anticoagulation regimen for AF was the use of VKA, also called coumarins. They included acenocoumarol, phenprocoumon, fluindione, and warfarin [37]. Warfarin is by far the most common of these and is the most commonly used anticoagulant [38]. These are effective agents, but they have certain disadvantages: a narrow therapeutic range, required laboratory monitoring, good patient adherence for safety and effectiveness, and certain risks for drug-drug and drug-food interactions [39].

The emergence of NOAC drugs has changed the paradigm for anticoagulation therapy. These agents have been shown noninferior to warfarin with respect to thromboembolism. They may alleviate some of the disadvantages of VKA anticoagulation, but some of them do not have reversal agents. A short summary of anticoagulants appears in **Table 3**.

	Apixaban	Dabigatran	Edoxaban	Rivaroxaban	Warfarin
Dosing	5 mg × 2 but 2.5 mg × 2 if two of the following: age > 80 years, weight < 60 kg, or creatinine >133 μmol/l	150 mg × 2 or 110 mg × 2 if either: age > 80 h, GFR 30–50 ml/min, GI disease, increased risk of bleeding	60 mg × 1 but 30 × 1 if one of the following: weight ≤ 60 kg, concomitant ciclosporin, dronedarone, erythromycin, ketoconazole	20 mg × 1 but 15 mg × 1 if GFR 15–50 ml/min	Strat dose 5–7.5 mg, daily, and then adjustment to INR
Renal failure	Contraindicated	Contraindicated	Contraindicated	Contraindicated	Approved indication
Risk of intracranial bleeding vs. warfarin	Lower	Lower	Lower	Lower	—
Interactions with other drugs or food	Few	Few but note dronedarone	Few	Few	Numerous
Possible to crush tablet	Yes	No	Yes	Yes	Yes
Independent of timing of food intake	Yes	Yes	Yes	No	Yes
Laboratory follow-up	6–12 months	6–12 months	6–12 months	6–12 months	Frequent, typically 1–2 every month
Specific antidote	No	Yes, instant effect	No	No	Yes, slow effect

Table 3.
A short summary of anticoagulation agents.

5.1 Vitamin K antagonists

Vitamin K antagonists (VKA) act by reducing the synthesis of the coagulation factors that rely on vitamin K. They inhibit the liver's ability to synthesize the precursors to clotting factors, Factor II (prothrombin), Factor VII, Factor IX, and Factor X. For that reason, it may take up to 2 weeks before all of these factors are eliminated and the drug is effective [35]. Warfarin may be reversed with oral or intravenous vitamin K, although the reversal may take hours to take effect [40]. Warfarin is an effective anticoagulant as long as blood concentrations fall within a relatively narrow therapeutic range; regular monitoring for time in therapeutic range is required. There is a wealth of clinical experience with VKA to inform prescribing choices.

Although warfarin may seem to be eclipsed by newer and more convenient agents, warfarin is still frequently prescribed and may be the optimal choice for some patients. VKA anticoagulation therapy decreases the risk of ischemic stroke in AF patients by >60%, although it does present a slightly increased risk for bleeding (<0.3%/year) [41].

Prescribing considerations for warfarin must include its narrow therapeutic index (overdosing may cause bleeding, and underdosing may cause thrombosis). Thus, warfarin patients must be followed with regular assessment of their international normalized ratio (INR). While genetics influence how an individual responds to VKA, such tests are not often used, and there is little guidance in terms of how to apply the findings from such genetic tests to therapeutic choices [42, 43]. Warfarin can be monitored at home with a home-based system and weekly test strips. The direct cost of warfarin is lower than for NOAC medications.

An important safety concern about warfarin involves hemorrhagic stroke which may occur in patients on VKA therapy. In fact, about 12–14% of cases of intracerebral hemorrhage are associated with warfarin [44]. VKA agents appear to contribute to vascular calcification to a greater extent than NOACs [45]. Drug-drug or food-drug interactions often occur with VKA therapy, particularly involving foods and drugs that induce or inhibit the CYP 450 enzymes [39, 46].

5.2 Non-vitamin-K antagonist oral anticoagulants (NOACs)

Four NOAC medications are approved and indicated for stroke prevention in patients with nonvalvular AF in the USA with some international variations. The NOAC category offers drugs in two classes: those that inhibit Factor Xa (apixaban, edoxaban, rivaroxaban) and direct thrombin inhibitors (dabigatran). Trials have demonstrated they are effective anticoagulation options with reasonable safety profiles. The advantages of NOACs compared to VKA therapy include predictable pharmacokinetics, rapid onset and offset of action, recent promising evidence from clinical trials showing reductions in stroke, intracranial hemorrhage, and all-cause mortality [46]. NOACs offer advantages, but the lingering concern with such medications is the lack of a reversal agent to stop the anticoagulatory effect in the event of a bleeding emergency for all these agents except dabigatran. The monoclonal antibody idarucizumab is available as a specific, with rapid onset, reversal agent for dabigatran [47].

5.2.1 Apixaban

Apixaban is a highly selective direct inhibitor of activated coagulation Factor X that can indirectly inhibit thrombin-induced platelet aggregation. It is an oral anticoagulant with linear and predictable pharmacokinetics and rapid onset/offset of action and has relatively few potential drug-drug or drug-food interactions [48]. In a meta-analysis of 16 studies, apixaban was more effective in reducing the rate of thromboembolic events compared to warfarin but similar to warfarin in reducing the risk of stroke [49]. However, it may reflect patient selection, and it is important to stress that no head-to-head studies with a randomized controlled have been conducted.

A post hoc analysis of the Apixaban for Reduction in Stroke and Other Thromboembolic Events in Atrial Fibrillation (ARISTOTLE) study compared clinical characteristics and outcomes in AF patients with a history of cancer taking either apixaban or warfarin. The outcomes were stroke, systemic embolism, major bleeding, and mortality [50]. In the study, 157 patients had active cancer, the remaining 1079 had remote cancer, and they were compared to 16,947 patients without cancer. No significant relationships between cancer and stroke, systemic embolism, ischemic stroke, or death could be determined, and the relationship between cancer and myocardial infarction was not significant after statistical adjustment. Apixaban was associated with improved rates of the composite endpoint (stroke, systemic embolism, myocardial infarction, and mortality) in those with active cancer and in those without cancer but not in those with remote cancer [50]. In a post hoc analysis of the ARISTOTLE study, 76.5% of patients were found to be on polypharmacy, defined as ≥5 or more drugs, and mortality, stroke, and systemic embolism rates increased with the greater number of concomitant medications [51]. Apixaban was deemed to be more effective than warfarin in AF patients on polypharmacy compared to warfarin and at least equivalent in terms of safety. An analysis of ARISTOTLE study data found 104 patients had a bioprosthetic heart valve replacement, and 52 had undergone valve repair. The safety and effectiveness of apixaban in this subpopulation was consistent with the larger study results, that is, apixaban may be an appropriate choice for a patient with valve replacement or repair [52]. Using data from this study, it was found that 30.5% of patients were taking potentially interacting medications at the time of the study (2722 apixaban and 2824 warfarin patients), which is common among AF patients. For the primary outcome endpoint (stroke or systemic embolism), both apixaban and warfarin were similar, and interacting medications had no effect on this outcome [53]. Apixaban results were also consistent in the multimorbid population (64% of ARISTOTLE population, defined as ≥3 comorbid conditions); apixaban was similarly effective in the general ARISTOTLE population as in the multimorbid subpopulations, including those with high multimorbidity (≥6 comorbid conditions) [54].

Using a Markov model and a population model from 2017 to 2030, apixaban was compared to warfarin in the German population of nonvalvular AF patients. The study showed that apixaban use instead of a VKA could avoid 52,185 major clinical events, including 14,319 all-cause deaths and 15,383 nonfatal strokes [55]. A Department of Defense study in the USA (n = 41,001) found apixaban was associated with a significantly lower risk of stroke, systemic embolism, or major bleeding compared to warfarin and to rivaroxaban [56].

5.2.2 Dabigatran

Dabigatran, a prodrug, is a direct thrombin inhibitor with predictable pharmacokinetics and pharmacodynamics, no need for laboratory monitoring, and fewer drug-food and drug-drug interactions compared to VKA. Unlike other NOAC drugs, dabigatran has an approved specific reversal agent, idarucizumab [57]. Dabigatran holds the distinction of being the first NOAC agent to be approved for nonvalvular AF patients [58].

The Randomized Evaluation of Long-Term Anticoagulant Therapy (RE-LY) study (n = 18,113) compared dabigatran at two doses (150 or 110 mg twice a day) to warfarin in a trial of AF patients that excluded those with mechanical heart valves, moderate to severe mitral stenosis, or valvular heart disease requiring intervention (patients with valvular heart disease not requiring intervention could be included) [59]. For dabigatran 150 mg twice daily, the rate of stroke or systemic embolic events was significantly lower than that of patients taking warfarin, but for those on 110 mg twice daily, rates were similar to warfarin. Intracranial bleed rates and mortality rates were significantly lower in both dabigatran groups compared to warfarin regardless of whether or not the patient had valvular heart disease [59].

The randomized phase II study to evaluate the safety and pharmacokinetics of oral dabigatran etexilate in patients after heart valve replacement (RE-ALIGN) study was terminated early when it compared VKA therapy to dabigatran and the dabigatran group experienced a high rate of thromboembolic and bleeding adverse events [60]. The study enrolled patients undergoing atrial and/or mitral mechanical valve implantation who were administered with 150 or 300 mg of dabigatran twice a day to determine relative safety and effectiveness of dabigatran compared to warfarin [61]. Dabigatran patients experienced higher rates of adverse events: 5% had strokes, 2% transient ischemic attacks, and 2% myocardial infarction compared to only transient ischemic attacks only at a rate of 2% in the warfarin group. The reasons for this have been speculated: dabigatran doses were too high, dabigatran was introduced too soon after valve surgery, or there remain factors to be elucidated about thromboembolic risks associated with artificial heart valves [62].

5.2.3 Edoxaban

Edoxaban, a factor Xa inhibitor, is approved for the prevention of stroke in nonvalvular AF patients. Factor Xa is a protease that serves to convert prothrombin into thrombin which, in turn, converts fibrinogen into fibrin and allows for clotting. Edoxaban has a dual mechanism of action in that it inhibits both free Factor Xa and also the by-product Factor Xa produced by prothrombinase [63]. Like other NOAC medications, it requires less laboratory monitoring, has fewer drug-drug and food-drug interactions, and lowers the risk of major bleeding compared to warfarin. It is not metabolized via the CYP450 enzyme system (which is the case for apixaban and rivaroxaban), and it was shown in the ENGAGE AF-TIMI study to be noninferior to warfarin. It is an oral agent that need be taken only once daily [63]. The safety and efficacy of edoxaban seem to be similar to other NOAC medications for the control of venous thromboembolism to reduce the risk of stroke in nonvalvular AF patients.

The Effective Anticoagulation with Factor Xa Next Generation in Atrial Fibrillation-Thrombosis in Myocardial Infarction 48 study (ENGAGE-AF-TIMI 48) compared edoxaban to warfarin in AF patients with and without valvular heart disease [64]. Valvular heart disease is associated with an increased risk for major adverse cardiovascular events, major bleeding, and death. Higher-dose edoxaban was found to be similarly effective to warfarin for all endpoints (stroke, systemic embolic event, major bleeding) in a trial of 18,222 patients [64].

A substudy of ENGAGE AF-TIMI 48 examined the effect of patient age on bleeding risk (risk is greater with older age) and favored edoxaban over warfarin for AF patients ≥75 years [65]. As such, edoxaban may be preferred over warfarin in elderly patients at risk for falls [66].

5.2.4 Rivaroxaban

Rivaroxaban is an NOAC that acts as a selective, direct inhibitor of activated coagulation Factor Xa. It is an oral medication with a rapid onset/offset of action and short half-life. It does not require laboratory monitoring and has predictable pharmacokinetics and pharmacodynamics and relatively few drug-drug and drug-food interactions compared to warfarin [67]. There is currently no approved reversal agent for rivaroxaban.

The ROCKET-AF study (n = 14,264) compared rivaroxaban to warfarin and found rivaroxaban had a 1.7% risk of stroke or systemic embolism at 1 year compared to 2.2% for warfarin. The composite safety endpoint was major bleeding or major bleeding plus clinically relevant non-major bleeding and occurred at a rate of 14.9% for rivaroxaban and 14.5% for warfarin patients [68]. The study concluded that rivaroxaban was noninferior to warfarin in prevention of stroke and systemic embolism. There was no significant difference in major or non-major but clinically relevant bleeding between rivaroxaban and warfarin. Gastrointestinal bleeding occurred more often in rivaroxaban than warfarin patients, but rates of major bleeding were similar.

5.3 Rotation of anticoagulation

There may be cases when it becomes necessary to change from warfarin to an NOAC or vice versa. In the case of moving from VKA to an NOAC, INR monitoring is needed throughout the shift [14]. The opposite transition, from NOAC to VKA, may require bridging to heparin or starting off with a lower dose of the NOAC medication at first, INR twice a week (minimum), and adjustment of VKA until the INR reaches ≤2.0 [69].

5.4 Risks of anticoagulation

In an elderly population (262,611 patients ≥60 years free of dementia and stroke), it was observed that incident AF was associated with an increased risk of dementia independent of stroke, while anticoagulation therapy decreased the risk for dementia [70]. The association between AF and dementia is not well elucidated, but white matter lesions, silent brain infarcts, and microbleeds in the brain are more common in AF patients, and it is not clear whether anticoagulation might play a role in this decreased risk for dementia [71].

Patients with liver disease are at risk for increased bleeding with anticoagulation therapy (but not increased thromboembolic events) [72]. However, NOAC therapy was shown in a clinical study (n = 39) to be safe and effective in cirrhosis patients [73].

Warfarin is teratogenic and should not be administered to pregnant women or women of childbearing potential without a clear understanding that they must not get pregnant while taking this drug [74].

6. Emergency anticoagulation and emergency anticoagulation reversal

NOAC anticoagulation offers advantages over VKA anticoagulation but also poses new challenges in the management of emergency situations. Emergency thrombolysis for treatment of ischemic stroke requires that the coagulation system be intact and, for this reason, is contraindicated in patients taking NOAC drugs, unless the agent is completely reversed before [75]. Prothrombin time and other laboratory tests are often faster and easier to accomplish with VKA therapy than NOAC in emergencies. For major bleeding events, rapid reversal of anticoagulation may be required which is likewise easier with VKA; however, reversing VKA agents such as warfarin may still take hours. Among the NOAC options, only dabigatran has a reversal agent, while the reversal agents for the other NOAC medications are in development.

7. Evidence from clinical trials

The NOAC medications and warfarin have been the subject of large published clinical trials, but head-to-head studies among the NOACs have not yet been carried out, and attempts to analyze data across trials have been challenged by differences in study methodologies, the AF populations evaluated, definitions (stroke, AF, major bleeding, and so on), and composite endpoints [76]. A meta-analysis (n = 17 studies) comparing rivaroxaban, dabigatran, and warfarin in real-world settings found that rivaroxaban was similar to warfarin in terms of the risks for major bleeding, myocardial infarction, and all-cause mortality; rivaroxaban was associated with a lower risk for stroke or systemic thromboembolism compared to warfarin; however, rivaroxaban had a higher risk for gastrointestinal bleeding than warfarin. Compared to dabigatran, rivaroxaban had similar risks for stroke and systemic thromboembolism and myocardial infarction, but the risks for major bleeding, gastrointestinal bleeding, and all-cause mortality were higher with rivaroxaban than dabigatran [77]. A retrospective study found that rivaroxaban and apixaban elevate the INR to levels above the high cutoff for normal (84.2% of rivaroxaban and 78.3% of apixaban with rivaroxaban significantly higher than apixaban, $p < 0.001$); however the clinical implications for these elevated INR values are not known [78].

A retrospective study of 1365 geriatric patients with head trauma found that NOAC therapy was a safer alternative than warfarin, although warfarin and NOACs were associated with similar mortality rates. NOAC patients had a lower rate of intracranial hemorrhage progression [79]. A retrospective database study of nonvalvular AF patients newly started on rivaroxaban, apixaban, or warfarin matched 11,411 rivaroxaban users to 11,411 warfarin patients and reported that the risk of ischemic stroke or intracranial hemorrhage was significantly lower in the rivaroxaban patients than in the warfarin patients. The study further matched 4083 apixaban patients to 4083 warfarin patients and found the combined endpoint (ischemic stroke or intracranial hemorrhage) was nonsignificantly reduced by apixaban versus warfarin. Apixaban reduced the risk of intracranial hemorrhage (hazard ratio 0.38, 95% confidence interval, 0.17–0.88) compared to warfarin, but the risk of ischemic stroke was nonsignificantly increased by apixaban versus warfarin (hazard ratio 1.13, 95% confidence interval, 0.49–2.63). The study did not compare rivaroxaban to apixaban [80].

In a study of 962 consecutive TAVR patients prescribed with NOAC (n = 326) or VKA therapy (n = 636) after surgery, the composite study endpoint were all-cause mortality, myocardial infarction, and any cerebrovascular event. After 1 year of follow-up from TAVR, the composite endpoint occurred in 21.2% of NOAC and 15.0% of VKA patients. Rates of bleeding and all-cause mortality were similar, but NOACs had a higher rate of ischemic events than VKA therapy [81]. In a systematic review of anticoagulation therapy in AF patients with valvular heart disease and bioprosthetic heart valves, edoxaban 30 mg was associated with the least rate of major bleeding compared to rivaroxaban, VKA, and other similar agents. Overall, NOAC medications were more effective in this population than warfarin, and NOACs were similar with the exception of edoxaban and major bleeding rates [82].

Evidence from clinical trials shows promise but does not yet provide clinicians with a complete picture. For example, patients with moderate to severe mitral stenosis or those with a mechanical heart valve are both at elevated risk from thromboembolism and typically excluded from head-to-head clinical trials that compare VKAs to specific NOACs. There are also patient groups who have been included in some, but not other trials, for example, patients who had a previous heart valve surgery (but not a mechanical valve) were excluded from RE-LY but included in ROCKET-AF, ARISTOTLE, and ENGAGE-AF. Patients with AF and a mechanical heart valve are routinely excluded from most head-to-head trials on anticoagulation. Thus, there are gaps in the evidence as to which types of anticoagulation treatments are most effective in specific populations.

8. Clinical considerations for oral anticoagulants

Although it is well known that anticoagulation therapy can help prevent stroke in AF patients at risk for thromboembolic events, only about half of the indicated patients actually are prescribed with therapy [83]. There is an inverse relationship between antiplatelet prescription and non-prescription of anticoagulation therapy. However, antiplatelet therapy is not as effective as anticoagulation medications for stroke prevention [84]. When prescribing anticoagulation therapy, the clinician must evaluate several factors: the indications for anticoagulation therapy, individual patient characteristics, whether or not the patient is taking other medications, patient preferences (if any), clinician and institutional preferences, and cost [14]. When antiplatelet therapy is combined with anticoagulation, the risk for bleeding increases [14]. Among patients with nonvalvular AF, those with heart failure and/or left-ventricular dysfunction have higher rates of bleeding and stroke/systemic embolism. Although some large trials of NOACs have included such patients, there have been no specific studies to investigate the safety of such drugs in these populations [85], and there is little evidence to guide prescribing choices.

Comorbidities must be considered when selecting the optimal anticoagulation regimen for a specific patient. Hepatic disease may increase the patient's risk for bleeding and impairs hepatic drug metabolism and clearance. In NOAC trials, patients with liver disease were excluded, so there is a paucity of evidence about how to use NOAC therapy in this population. A retrospective database study from Korea (12,778 warfarin patients and 24,575 NOAC patients) found NOACs reduced the risk for ischemic stroke, intracranial hemorrhage, gastrointestinal bleeding, major bleeding, and all-cause death compared to warfarin. In the 13% of this study population with active liver disease, there was a lower rate for the composite endpoint (all endpoints above) for NOAC than warfarin [86].

Renal failure, common in AF patients, has an inflammatory pathophysiology and puts patients at risk for both thromboembolitic events and bleeding [87]. Since NOACs are cleared by the kidneys, renal failure has an adverse effect on NOAC pharmacokinetics but not on warfarin. However, warfarin likewise can interact with other drugs including drugs taken by patients managing kidney disorders [88]. A retrospective database study in Germany, RELOAD, compared outcomes of nonvalvular AF patients with compromised renal function taking either rivaroxaban or phenprocoumon (VKA therapy) and found that for patients with no evidence of cancer, rivaroxaban was associated with a lower rate of ischemic stroke and intracranial hemorrhage compared to phenprocoumon [89]. Warfarin is also more commonly prescribed to nonvalvular AF patients on hemodialysis, and while no head-to-head clinical trials have compared warfarin to NOACs in this population, dialysis patients are sometimes prescribed with NOAC therapy. The preference for NOACs in the hemodialysis population may be due to several concerns: it is difficult to maintain warfarin at INR in the therapeutic range, warfarin may calcify vasculature, and dialysis patients have an elevated risk of intracranial hemorrhage. Hemodialysis patients are challenging for anticoagulation, because they often are multimorbid, have extensive antibiotic exposure, and may have vitamin K deficiency. Adherence can also be especially problematic in the hemodialysis population [90].

The role of anticoagulation in cancer patients becomes complex as many cancer patients are at increased bleeding risk and may be taking antiplatelet agents and nonsteroidal anti-inflammatory drugs, have renal impairment, or be on chemotherapy. Many chemotherapeutic agents increase the patient's risk of arterial and venous thrombosis, and chemotherapy that induces thrombocytopenia may elevate bleeding risks [91]. There is also the risk that anticoagulants may interact with chemotherapeutic agents or supportive-care drugs. Many chemotherapeutic regimens (cisplatin, melphalan, cyclophosphamide) and some monoclonal antibodies increase the risk of nonvalvular AF. Cancer patients with AF have an increased risk for thromboembolism [92]. There is only limited knowledge of the risk of ischemic stroke attributable to cancer, and many risk assessment tools do not incorporate cancer. Further, cancer is not just one disease, and there may be important clinical variations with respect to the type of cancer, AF risk, and risk of thromboembolism and stroke [93].

Patient factors may also influence prescribing choices. Patient adherence must be considered in long-term anticoagulation therapy; the continuously adherent rate is under 45% for those newly diagnosed AF patients prescribed with some form of anticoagulation therapy [94]. Patient education may play a role in improving adherence. In a study of 339 adults on anticoagulation treatment for nonvalvular AF, participants evidenced moderate knowledge about AF but had a more limited understanding of anticoagulation and stroke [95]. Thus, better educational efforts may be helpful. Culture and ethnicity may also be a consideration when making prescribing determinations. In a multinational survey of 937 adults on anticoagulation treatment for nonvalvular AF, national differences emerged such that US patients perceived AF as a serious condition, whereas the Japanese were less concerned about AF, but both were quite concerned about stroke risks. French patients preferred the physician to select AF therapy, while German, US, and Canadian patients preferred to be involved in therapeutic choices [96]. A cross-sectional survey of 226 physician specialists in Bulgaria also reports that 68% of patients who have an indication for anticoagulation therapy preferred a shared decision-making approach, and only 19% wanted the physician to make all anticoagulation therapy choices [97]. Improved understanding about the risk of stroke, the nature of stroke, and anticoagulation treatment may improve adherence and empower patients in their own care.

Women taking warfarin have a greater risk of stroke/embolism than men, but this sex difference is not maintained for all of the NOACs [98]. Moreover, there is some evidence that with NOACs, women have less risk of major bleeding than men. The differences have been discussed in the literature and do not seem to apply to anticoagulation effectiveness [99]. Further studies are needed, but it appears that NOAC drugs may have some sex-based differences that at this time seem clinically unimportant.

9. Device-based approaches

Some patients have a relative or absolute contraindication to anticoagulation therapy. Device-based approaches may be important options for these patients.

It exceeds the scope of this chapter to describe these devices, their implantation, and results in detail, but a brief introduction is offered. Direct closure of the LAA via a minimally invasive surgical procedure is well established. It is a safe, effective procedure that can generally be performed in 30–40 min. Initially, the LAA was closed utilizing an endoscopic stapler, but more recently a minimally invasive LAA surgical clip is used (AtriClip, AtriCure, Inc., Cincinnati, Ohio, USA). The clip offers complete closure immediately, and no postoperative anticoagulation is needed.

A device implanted under fluoroscopic control into the orifice of the LAA by transseptal puncture may also be used (Watchman, Boston Scientific, Inc., Boston, Massachusetts, USA). This device has a high leak rate, and the US Food and Drug Administration requires postoperative anticoagulation for several weeks after implantation. Five-year outcomes from two large randomized clinical trials (PREVAIL and PROTECT AF) found that LAA closure with the WATCHMAN device offered stroke prevention in patients with nonvalvular AF comparable to that of warfarin with additional reductions in major bleeding and mortality [100].

In contrast to these is a suture-based occluding device (Lariat, SentreHEART, Redwood City, California, USA) that requires transseptal implantation. Unlike WATCHMAN, this device does in fact close the LAA, but in addition to a transseptal puncture, it requires access to the pericardium. A large randomized multicenter controlled trial is ongoing to determine the 30-day safety of this device and freedom from documented episodes of AF, atrial flutter, or atrial tachycardia >30 s at 12 months with a secondary composite endpoint of cardiovascular death or stroke [101].

10. Conclusions

New anticoagulation therapies are changing the paradigm of anticoagulation treatment for patients with certain forms of AF. This shift is further complicated by the fact that the definition and understanding of nonvalvular versus valvular AF are under scrutiny and evolving. Vitamin K antagonism (warfarin and other drugs) had been the standard of care for decades and still represents an important anticoagulation option. The main drawbacks to VKA are the need for laboratory monitoring and strict therapy adherence to maintain anticoagulation efficacy plus the potential for drug-drug and food-drug interactions. A benefit for warfarin and other VKA treatments is the fact that the anticoagulation effect can be pharmacologically reversed. The arrival of the NOAC agents presents improved effectiveness in many key endpoints such as stroke prevention and similar or enhanced safety with respect to bleeding risks. There are four of these drugs (apixaban, dabigatran, edoxaban, and rivaroxaban), but as yet there are no head-to-head clinical trials among them for clinical guidance. Except for dabigatran, there are presently no reversal agents for these drugs. Clinicians must evaluate these anticoagulation approaches to make individualized decisions for patients. Further study is needed, particularly for specific subpopulations of AF patients: those with heart failure, implanted devices, renal compromise, and cancer.

Conflicts of interest

Peter Magnusson has received speaker fees or grants from Abbott, Alylam, Bayer, AstraZeneca, BMS, Boeringer-Ingelheim, Lilly, Novo Nordisk, Octupus

Medical, and Pfizer. Joseph Pergolizzi is a principal at Native Cardio, Inc. Randall K. Wolf is a paid consultant to the engineering team at AtriCure, Inc. Morten Lamberts has received speaker fees from BMS. Jo Ann LeQuang has no relevant disclosures.

Author details

Peter Magnusson[1,2], Joseph V. Pergolizzi Jr [3,4], Randall K. Wolf[5], Morten Lamberts[6] and Jo Ann LeQuang[3*]

1 Centre for Research and Development, Uppsala/Region, Gävleborg, Gävle, Sweden

2 Department of Medicine, Cardiology Research Unit, Karolinska Institutet, Stockholm, Sweden

3 NEMA Research, Inc., Naples, Florida, USA

4 Native Cardio, Inc., Naples, Florida, USA

5 DeBakey Heart and Vascular Center, Houston Methodist Hospital, Texas Medical Center, Houston, Texas, USA

6 Department of Cardiology, Herlev-Gentofte University Hospital, Copenhagen, Denmark

*Address all correspondence to: joannlequang@gmail.com

References

[1] Lin H-J, Wolf P, Kelly-Hayes M, Beiser A, Kase C, Benjamin E, et al. Stroke severity in atrial fibrillation: The Framngham Study. Stroke. 1996;**27**:1760-1764

[2] Amerena J, Ridley D. An update on anticoagulation in atrial fibrillation. Heart, Lung & Circulation. 2017;**26**(9):911-917

[3] Fauchier L, Philippart R, Clementy N, Bourguignon T, Angoulvant D, Ivanes F, et al. How to define valvular atrial fibrillation? Archives of Cardiovascular Diseases. 2015;**108**(10):530-539

[4] Kirchhof P, Benussi S, Kotecha D, Ahlsson A, Atar D, Casadei B, et al. 2016 ESC Guidelines for the management of atrial fibrillation developed in collaboration with EACTS. Europace: European Pacing, Arrhythmias, and Cardiac Electrophysiology: Journal of the Working Groups on Cardiac Pacing, Arrhythmias, and Cardiac Cellular Electrophysiology of the European Society of Cardiology. 2016;**18**(11):1609-1678

[5] January CT, Wann LS, Alpert JS, Calkins H, Cigarroa JE, Cleveland JC Jr, et al. 2014 AHA/ACC/HRS guideline for the management of patients with atrial fibrillation: A report of the American College of Cardiology/American Heart Association Task Force on Practice Guidelines and the Heart Rhythm Society. Journal of the American College of Cardiology. 2014;**64**(21):e1-e76

[6] Doherty JU, Gluckman TJ, Hucker WJ, Januzzi JL Jr, Ortel TL, Saxonhouse SJ, et al. 2017 ACC expert consensus decision pathway for periprocedural management of anticoagulation in patients with nonvalvular atrial fibrillation: A report of the American College of Cardiology Clinical Expert Consensus Document Task Force. Journal of the American College of Cardiology. 2017;**69**(7):871-898

[7] Lip GYH, Banerjee A, Boriani G, Chiang CE, Fargo R, Freedman B, et al. Antithrombotic therapy for atrial fibrillation: CHEST guideline and expert panel report. Chest. 2018;**154**(5):1121-1201

[8] Macle L, Cairns J, Leblanc K, Tsang T, Skanes A, Cox JL, et al. 2016 focused update of the Canadian cardiovascular society guidelines for the management of atrial fibrillation. The Canadian Journal of Cardiology. 2016;**32**(10):1170-1185

[9] Andrade JG, Verma A, Mitchell LB, Parkash R, Leblanc K, Atzema C, et al. 2018 focused update of the Canadian cardiovascular society guidelines for the management of atrial fibrillation. The Canadian journal of cardiology. 2018;**34**(11):1371-1392

[10] De Caterina R, John Camm A. Non-vitamin K antagonist oral anticoagulants in atrial fibrillation accompanying mitral stenosis: The concept for a trial. Europace: European Pacing, Arrhythmias, and Cardiac Electrophysiology: Journal of the Working Groups on Cardiac Pacing, Arrhythmias, and Cardiac Cellular Electrophysiology of the European Society of Cardiology. 2016;**18**(1):6-11

[11] Lip GYH, Collet JP, de Caterina R, Fauchier L, Lane DA, Larsen TB, et al. Antithrombotic Therapy in Atrial Fibrillation Associated with valvular Heart Disease: Executive Summary of a Joint Consensus Document from the European Heart Rhythm Association (EHRA) and European Society of Cardiology Working Group on Thrombosis, Endorsed by the ESC Working Group on valvular Heart Disease, Cardiac Arrhythmia Society

of Southern Africa (CASSA), Heart Rhythm Society (HRS), Asia Pacific Heart Rhythm Society (APHRS), South African Heart (SA Heart) Association and Sociedad Latinoamericana de Estimulacion Cardiaca y Electrofisiologia (SOLEACE). Thrombosis and Haemostasis. 2017;**117**(12):2215-2236

[12] Brieger D, Amerena J, Attia J, Bajorek B, Chan KH, Connell C, et al. National Heart Foundation of Australia and the Cardiac Society of Australia and New Zealand: Australian Clinical Guidelines for the Diagnosis and Management of Atrial Fibrillation 2018. Heart, Lung & Circulation. 2018;**27**(10):1209-1266

[13] Vedovati MC, Reboldi G, Agnelli G, Verdecchia P. Type 2 valvular heart disease affects decision making for anticoagulation in patients with atrial fibrillation: The UMBRIA-fibrillazione atriale prospective study. TH Open: Companion Journal to Thrombosis and Haemostasis. 2019;**3**(2):e157-ee64

[14] Kovacs RJ, Flaker GC, Saxonhouse SJ, Doherty JU, Birtcher KK, Cuker A, et al. Practical management of anticoagulation in patients with atrial fibrillation. Journal of the American College of Cardiology. 2015;**65**(13):1340-1360

[15] Nkomo VT, Gardin JM, Skelton TN, Gottdiener JS, Scott CG, Enriquez-Sarano M. Burden of valvular heart diseases: A population-based study. Lancet (London, England). 2006;**368**(9540):1005-1011

[16] Angiolillo DJ, Pineda AM. Oral anticoagulation after TAVR in patients with atrial fibrillation. The Certainty of Uncertainty. JACC Cardiovascular Interventions. 2019;**12**(16):1577-1579

[17] Sherwood MW, Vora AN. Challenges in aortic stenosis: Review of antiplatelet/anticoagulant therapy management with transcatheter aortic valve replacement (TAVR): TAVR with recent PCI, TAVR in the patient with atrial fibrillation, and TAVR thrombosis management. Current Cardiology Reports. 2018;**20**(12):130

[18] Sherwood MW, Vemulapalli S, Harrison JK, Dai D, Vora AN, Mack MJ, et al. Variation in post-TAVR antiplatelet therapy utilization and associated outcomes: Insights from the STS/ACC TVT registry. American Heart Journal. 2018;**204**:9-16

[19] Megaly M, Garcia S, Anzia LE, Morley P, Garberich R, Gornick CC, et al. Detection of atrial fibrillation and atrial flutter by pacemaker device interrogation after transcatheter aortic valve replacement (TAVR): Implications for management. The Journal of Invasive Cardiology. 2019;**31**(7):E177-E183

[20] Di Biase L, Burkhardt JD, Santangeli P, Mohanty P, Sanchez JE, Horton R, et al. Periprocedural stroke and bleeding complications in patients undergoing catheter ablation of atrial fibrillation with different anticoagulation management: Results from the role of coumadin in preventing thromboembolism in atrial fibrillation (AF) patients undergoing catheter ablation (COMPARE) randomized trial. Circulation. 2014;**129**(25):2638-2644

[21] Lakkireddy D, Reddy YM, Di Biase L, Vanga SR, Santangeli P, Swarup V, et al. Feasibility and safety of dabigatran versus warfarin for periprocedural anticoagulation in patients undergoing radiofrequency ablation for atrial fibrillation: Results from a multicenter prospective registry. Journal of the American College of Cardiology. 2012;**59**(13):1168-1174

[22] Kim JS, She F, Jongnarangsin K, Chugh A, Latchamsetty R, Ghanbari H, et al. Dabigatran vs

warfarin for radiofrequency catheter ablation of atrial fibrillation. Heart Rhythm. 2013;**10**(4):483-489

[23] Providencia R, Albenque JP, Combes S, Bouzeman A, Casteigt B, Combes N, et al. Safety and efficacy of dabigatran versus warfarin in patients undergoing catheter ablation of atrial fibrillation: A systematic review and meta-analysis. Heart (British Cardiac Society). 2014;**100**(4):324-335

[24] Calkins H, Willems S, Gerstenfeld EP, Verma A, Schilling R, Hohnloser SH, et al. Uninterrupted dabigatran versus warfarin for ablation in atrial fibrillation. The New England Journal of Medicine. 2017;**376**(17):1627-1636

[25] Kirchhof P, Haeusler KG, Blank B, De Bono J, Callans D, Elvan A, et al. Apixaban in patients at risk of stroke undergoing atrial fibrillation ablation. European Heart Journal. 2018;**39**(32):2942-2955

[26] Cappato R, Marchlinski FE, Hohnloser SH, Naccarelli GV, Xiang J, Wilber DJ, et al. Uninterrupted rivaroxaban vs. uninterrupted vitamin K antagonists for catheter ablation in non-valvular atrial fibrillation. European Heart Journal. 2015;**36**(28):1805-1811

[27] Birnie DH, Healey JS, Wells GA, Verma A, Tang AS, Krahn AD, et al. Pacemaker or defibrillator surgery without interruption of anticoagulation. The New England Journal of Medicine. 2013;**368**(22):2084-2093

[28] Rho R, Page R. Asymptomatic atrial fibrillation. Progress in Cardiovascular Diseases. 2005;**48**:79-87

[29] Sandgren E, Rorsman C, Edvardsson N, Engdahl J. Stroke incidence and anticoagulation treatment in patients with pacemaker-detected silent atrial fibrillation. PLoS One. 2018;**13**(9):e0203661

[30] Smith EE, Saposnik G, Biessels GJ, Doubal FN, Fornage M, Gorelick PB, et al. Prevention of stroke in patients with silent cerebrovascular disease: A scientific statement for healthcare professionals from the American Heart Association/American Stroke Association. Stroke. 2017;**48**(2):e44-e71

[31] Hahne K, Monnig G, Samol A. Atrial fibrillation and silent stroke: Links, risks, and challenges. Vascular Health and Risk Management. 2016;**12**:65-74

[32] Deneke T, Jais P, Scaglione M, Schmitt R, DIB L, Christopoulos G, et al. Silent cerebral events/lesions related to atrial fibrillation ablation: A clinical review. Journal of Cardiovascular Electrophysiology. 2015;**26**(4):455-463

[33] Friberg L, Skeppholm M, Terent A. Benefit of anticoagulation unlikely in patients with atrial fibrillatio and a CHA2DS2-VASc score of 1. Journal of the American College of Cardiology. 2015;**65**:225-232

[34] Chao TF, Wang KL, Liu CJ, Lin YJ, Chang SL, Lo LW, et al. Age threshold for increased stroke risk among patients with atrial fibrillation: A nationwide cohort study from Taiwan. Journal of the American College of Cardiology. 2015;**66**(12):1339-1347

[35] Fender AC, Dobrev D. Anticoagulation in difficult settings RELOADed: Evidence for applicability of direct oral anticoagulants in patients with atrial fibrillation, renal impairment and cancer. International Journal of Cardiology Heart & Vasculature. 2019;**23**:100374

[36] Pisters R, Lane DA, Nieuwlaat R, de Vos CB, Crijns HJ, Lip GY. A novel user-friendly score (HAS-BLED) to assess 1-year risk of major bleeding in patients with atrial fibrillation: The Euro Heart Survey. Chest. 2010;**138**(5):1093-1100

[37] Wardrop D, Keeling D. The story of the discovery of heparin and warfarin. British Journal of Haematology. 2008;**141**:757-763

[38] Pirmohamed M. Warfarin: Almost 60 years old and still causing problems. British Journal of Clinical Pharmacology. 2006;**62**:509-511

[39] Norwood DA, Parke CK, Rappa LR. A comprehensive review of potential warfarin-fruit interactions. Journal of Pharmacy Practice. 2015;**28**(6):561-571

[40] Lubetsky A, Yonath H, Olchovsky D, Loebstein R, Halkin H, Ezra D. Comparison of oral vs intravenous phytonadione (vitamin K1) in patients with excessive anticoagulation: A prospective randomized controlled study. Archives of Internal Medicine. 2003;**163**(20):2469-2473

[41] Hart RG, Pearce LA, Aguilar MI. Meta-analysis: Antithrombotic therapy to prevent stroke in patients who have nonvalvular atrial fibrillation. Annals of Internal Medicine. 2007;**146**(12):857-867

[42] Pirmohamed M, Burnside G, Eriksson N, Jorgensen AL, Toh CH, Nicholson T, et al. A randomized trial of genotype-guided dosing of warfarin. The New England Journal of Medicine. 2013;**369**(24):2294-2303

[43] Kimmel SE, French B, Kasner SE, Johnson JA, Anderson JL, Gage BF, et al. A pharmacogenetic versus a clinical algorithm for warfarin dosing. The New England Journal of Medicine. 2013;**369**(24):2283-2293

[44] Radberg JA, Olsson JE, Radberg CT. Prognostic parameters in spontaneous intracerebral hematomas with special reference to anticoagulant treatment. Stroke. 1991;**22**(5):571-576

[45] Peeters F, Dudink E, Kimenai DM, Weijs B, Altintas S, Heckman LIB, et al. Vitamin K antagonists, non-vitamin K antagonist oral anticoagulants, and vascular calcification in patients with atrial fibrillation. TH Open: Companion Journal to Thrombosis and Haemostasis. 2018;**2**(4):e391-e398

[46] Delluc A, Wang TF, Yap ES, Ay C, Schaefer J, Carrier M, et al. Anticoagulation of cancer patients with non-valvular atrial fibrillation receiving chemotherapy: Guidance from the SSC of the ISTH. Journal of Thrombosis and Haemostasis. 2019;**17**(8):1247-1252

[47] Pollack CV Jr, Reilly PA, Weitz JI. Dabigatran reversal with idarucizumab. The New England Journal of Medicine. 2017;**377**(17):1691-1692

[48] Kubisz P, Stanciakova L, Dobrotova M, Samos M, Mokan M, Stasko J. Apixaban—Metabolism, pharmacologic properties and drug interactions. Current Drug Metabolism. 2017;**18**(7):609-621

[49] Proietti M, Romanazzi I, Romiti GF, Farcomeni A, Lip GYH. Real-world use of apixaban for stroke prevention in atrial fibrillation: A systematic review and meta-analysis. Stroke. 2018;**49**(1):98-106

[50] Melloni C, Dunning A, Granger CB, Thomas L, Khouri MG, Garcia DA, et al. Efficacy and safety of apixaban versus warfarin in patients with atrial fibrillation and a history of cancer: Insights from the ARISTOTLE Trial. The American Journal of Medicine. 2017;**130**(12):1440-1448.e1

[51] Jaspers Focks J, Brouwer MA, Wojdyla DM, Thomas L, Lopes RD, Washam JB, et al. Polypharmacy and effects of apixaban versus warfarin in patients with atrial fibrillation: Post hoc analysis of the ARISTOTLE trial. BMJ (Clinical Research Ed). 2016;**i2868**:353

[52] Guimaraes PO, Pokorney SD, Lopes RD, Wojdyla DM, Gersh BJ, Giczewska A, et al. Efficacy and safety

of apixaban vs warfarin in patients with atrial fibrillation and prior bioprosthetic valve replacement or valve repair: Insights from the ARISTOTLE trial. Clinical Cardiology. 2019;**42**(5):568-571

[53] Washam JB, Hohnloser SH, Lopes RD, Wojdyla DM, Vinereanu D, Alexander JH, et al. Interacting medication use and the treatment effects of apixaban versus warfarin: Results from the ARISTOTLE Trial. Journal of Thrombosis and Thrombolysis. 2019;**47**(3):345-352

[54] Alexander KP, Brouwer MA, Mulder H, Vinereanu D, Lopes RD, Proietti M, et al. Outcomes of apixaban versus warfarin in patients with atrial fibrillation and multi-morbidity: Insights from the ARISTOTLE trial. American Heart Journal. 2019;**208**:123-131

[55] Himmler S, Muller M, Ostwald D, Seddik A, Basic E, Hradetzky E. Long-term health benefits of stroke prevention with apixaban versus vitamin K antagonist warfarin in patients with non-valvular atrial fibrillation in Germany: A population-based modelling study. Expert Review of Pharmacoeconomics & Outcomes Research. 2019;**19**(2):223-230

[56] Gupta K, Trocio J, Keshishian A, Zhang Q, Dina O, Mardekian J, et al. Real-world comparative effectiveness, safety, and health care costs of oral anticoagulants in nonvalvular atrial fibrillation patients in the U.S. Department of Defense Population. Journal of Managed Care & Specialty Pharmacy. 2018;**24**(11):1116-1127

[57] Trailokya A, Hiremath JS. Dabigatran—The first approved DTI for SPAF. The Journal of the Association of Physicians of India. 2018;**66**(4):85-90

[58] Mumoli N, Mastroiacovo D, Tamborini-Permunian E, Vitale J, Giorgi-Pierfranceschi M, Cei M, et al. Dabigatran in nonvalvular atrial fibrillation: From clinical trials to real-life experience. Journal of cardiovascular medicine (Hagerstown, Md). 2017;**18**(7):467-477

[59] Ezekowitz MD, Nagarakanti R, Noack H, Brueckmann M, Litherland C, Jacobs M, et al. Comparison of dabigatran and warfarin in patients with atrial fibrillation and valvular heart disease: The RE-LY trial (randomized evaluation of long-term anticoagulant therapy). Circulation. 2016;**134**(8):589-598

[60] Eikelboom JW, Connolly SJ, Brueckmann M, Granger CB, Kappetein AP, Mack MJ, et al. Dabigatran versus warfarin in patients with mechanical heart valves. The New England Journal of Medicine. 2013;**369**(13):1206-1214

[61] Van de Werf F, Brueckmann M, Connolly SJ, Friedman J, Granger CB, Hartter S, et al. A comparison of dabigatran etexilate with warfarin in patients with mechanical heart valves: THE Randomized, phase II study to evaluate the safety and pharmacokinetics of oral dabigatran etexilate in patients after heart valve replacement (RE-ALIGN). American Heart Journal. 2012;**163**(6):931-937.e1

[62] Iung B, Vahanian A. Lessons from the RE-ALIGN trial. Archives of Cardiovascular Diseases. 2014;**107**(5):277-279

[63] Poulakos M, Walker JN, Baig U, David T. Edoxaban: A direct oral anticoagulant. American Journal of Health-System Pharmacy: AJHP: Official Journal of the American Society of Health-System Pharmacists. 2017;**74**(3):117-129

[64] De Caterina R, Renda G, Carnicelli AP, Nordio F, Trevisan M, Mercuri MF, et al. Valvular heart disease patients on edoxaban or warfarin in the ENGAGE AF-TIMI 48 trial. Journal of

the American College of Cardiology. 2017;**69**(11):1372-1382

[65] Kato ET, Giugliano RP, Ruff CT, Koretsune Y, Yamashita T, Kiss RG, et al. Efficacy and safety of edoxaban in elderly patients with atrial fibrillation in the ENGAGE AF-TIMI 48 trial. Journal of the American Heart Association. 2016;**5**(5):pii. E003432

[66] Steffel J, Giugliano RP, Braunwald E, Murphy SA, Mercuri M, Choi Y, et al. Edoxaban versus warfarin in atrial fibrillation patients at risk of falling: ENGAGE AF-TIMI 48 analysis. Journal of the American College of Cardiology. 2016;**68**(11):1169-1178

[67] Kvasnicka T, Malikova I, Zenahlikova Z, Kettnerova K, Brzezkova R, Zima T, et al. Rivaroxaban—Metabolism, pharmacologic properties and drug interactions. Current Drug Metabolism. 2017;**18**(7):636-642

[68] Patel MR, Mahaffey KW, Garg J, Pan G, Singer DE, Hacke W, et al. Rivaroxaban versus warfarin in nonvalvular atrial fibrillation. The New England Journal of Medicine. 2011;**365**(10):883-891

[69] Ruff CT, Giugliano RP, Braunwald E, Mercuri M, Curt V, Betcher J, et al. Transition of patients from blinded study drug to open-label anticoagulation: The ENGAGE AF-TIMI 48 trial. Journal of the American College of Cardiology. 2014;**64**(6):576-584

[70] Kim D, Yang PS, Yu HT, Kim TH, Jang E, Sung JH, et al. Risk of dementia in stroke-free patients diagnosed with atrial fibrillation: Data from a population-based cohort. European Heart Journal. 2019;**40**(28):2313-2323

[71] Demeestere J, Lemmens R. Anticoagulation in low-risk patients with atrial fibrillation: Beyond prevention of ischaemic stroke. European Heart Journal. 2019;**40**(28):2336-2338

[72] Qamar A, Antman EM, Ruff CT, Nordio F, Murphy SA, Grip LT, et al. Edoxaban versus warfarin in patients with atrial fibrillation and history of liver disease. Journal of the American College of Cardiology. 2019;**74**(2):179-189

[73] Intagliata NM, Henry ZH, Maitland H, Shah NL, Argo CK, Northup PG, et al. Direct oral anticoagulants in cirrhosis patients pose similar risks of bleeding when compared to traditional anticoagulation. Digestive Diseases and Sciences. 2016;**61**(6):1721-1727

[74] Conradie M, Henderson BD, Van Wyk C. Preventable warfarin-induced birth defects: A missed opportunity? South African Medical Journal = Suid-Afrikaanse tydskrif vir geneeskunde. 2019;**109**(6):415-420

[75] Diener HC, Foerch C, Riess H, Rother J, Schroth G, Weber R. Treatment of acute ischaemic stroke with thrombolysis or thrombectomy in patients receiving anti-thrombotic treatment. The Lancet Neurology. 2013;**12**(7):677-688

[76] Camm AJ, Fox KAA, Peterson E. Challenges in comparing the non-vitamin K antagonist oral anticoagulants for atrial fibrillation-related stroke prevention. Europace: European Pacing, Arrhythmias, and Cardiac Electrophysiology: Journal of the Working Groups on Cardiac Pacing, Arrhythmias, and Cardiac Cellular Electrophysiology of the European Society of Cardiology. 2018;**20**(1):1-11

[77] Bai Y, Deng H, Shantsila A, Lip GY. Rivaroxaban versus Dabigatran or warfarin in real-world studies of stroke prevention in atrial fibrillation: Systematic review and meta-analysis. Stroke. 2017;**48**(4):970-976

[78] Ofek F, Bar Chaim S, Kronenfeld N, Ziv-Baran T, Berkovitch M. International

normalized ratio is significantly elevated with rivaroxaban and apixaban drug therapies: A retrospective study. Clinical Therapeutics. 2017;**39**(5):1003-1010

[79] Scotti P, Seguin C, Lo BWY, de Guise E, Troquet JM, Marcoux J. Antithrombotic agents and traumatic brain injury in the elderly population: Hemorrhage patterns and outcomes. Journal of Neurosurgery. July 2019;**5**: 1-10. [Epub ahead of print]

[80] Coleman CI, Antz M, Bowrin K, Evers T, Simard EP, Bonnemeier H, et al. Real-world evidence of stroke prevention in patients with nonvalvular atrial fibrillation in the United States: The REVISIT-US study. Current Medical Research and Opinion. 2016;**32**(12):2047-2053

[81] Jochheim D, Barbanti M, Capretti G, Stefanini GG, Hapfelmeier A, Zadrozny M, et al. Oral anticoagulant type and outcomes AFTER TRANSCATheter aortic valve replacement. JACC Cardiovascular Interventions. 2019;**12**(16):1566-1576

[82] Malik AH, Yandrapalli S, Aronow WS, Panza JA, Cooper HA. Oral anticoagulants in atrial fibrillation with valvular heart disease and bioprosthetic heart valves. Heart (British Cardiac Society). 2019

[83] Piazza G, Karipineni N, Goldberg HS, Jenkins KL, Goldhaber SZ. Underutilization of anticoagulation for stroke prevention in atrial fibrillation. Journal of the American College of Cardiology. 2016;**67**(20):2444-2446

[84] Chopard R, Goldhaber SZ, Karipineni N, Goldberg HS, Piazza G. Antiplatelet prescription in atrial fibrillation: Association with a low rate of anticoagulation. TH Open: Companion Journal to Thrombosis and Haemostasis. 2018;**2**(2):e229-e232

[85] Chugh Y, Faillace RT. The C of CHADS: Historical perspective and clinical applications for anticoagulation in patients with non valvular atrial fibrillation and congestive heart failure. International Journal of Cardiology. 2016;**224**:431-436

[86] Lee SR, Lee HJ, Choi EK, Han KD, Jung JH, Cha MJ, et al. Direct oral anticoagulants in patients with atrial fibrillation and liver disease. Journal of the American College of Cardiology. 2019;**73**(25):3295-3308

[87] Ashish K, Bandyopadhyay D, Ghosh RK, Tan JL, Bose S. An intriguing relation between atrial fibrillation and contrast-induced nephropathy. International Journal of Cardiology Heart & Vasculature. 2018;**21**:78-79

[88] Fender AC, Dobrev D. Bound to bleed: How altered albumin binding may dictate warfarin treatment outcome. International Journal of Cardiology Heart & Vasculature. 2019;**22**:214-215

[89] Bonnemeier H, Huelsebeck M, Kloss S. Comparative effectiveness of rivaroxaban versus a vitamin K antagonist in patients with renal impairment treated for non-valvular atrial fibrillation in Germany—A retrospective cohort study. International Journal of Cardiology Heart & Vasculature. 2019;**23**:100367

[90] Reilly RF, Jain N. Warfarin in nonvalvular atrial fibrillation-time for a change? Seminars in Dialysis. 17 June 2019. DOI: 10.1111/sdi.12829. [Epub ahead of print]

[91] Avvisati G, Tirindelli MC, Annibali O. Thrombocytopenia and hemorrhagic risk in cancer patients. Critical Reviews in Oncology/Hematology. 2003;**48**(Suppl):S13-S16

[92] Hu Y, Liu C, Chang P, Taso H, Lin Y, Chang S, et al. Incident

thromboembolism and heart failure associated with new-onset atrial fibrillation in cancer patients. International Journal of Cardiology. 2013;**165**(2):355-357

[93] Navi BB, Reiner AS, Kamel H, Iadecola C, Okin PM, Elkind MSV, et al. Risk of arterial thromboembolism in patients with cancer. Journal of the American College of Cardiology. 2017;**70**(8):926-938

[94] Hernandez I, He M, Chen N, Brooks MM, Saba S, Gellad WF. Trajectories of oral anticoagulation adherence among medicare beneficiaries newly diagnosed with atrial fibrillation. Journal of the American Heart Association. 2019;**8**(12):e011427

[95] LaRosa AR, Pusateri AM, Althouse AD, Mathier AS, Essien UR, Magnani JW. Mind the gap: Deficits in fundamental disease-specific knowledge in atrial fibrillation. International Journal of Cardiology. 2019;**292**:272-276

[96] Lane DA, Meyerhoff J, Rohner U, Lip GYH. Patients' perceptions of atrial fibrillation, stroke risk, and oral anticoagulation treatment: An international survey. TH Open: Companion Journal to Thrombosis and Haemostasis. 2018;**2**(3):e233-e241

[97] Runev N, Potpara T, Naydenov S, Vladimirova A, Georgieva G, Manov E. Physicians' perceptions of their patients' attitude and knowledge of long-term oral anticoagulant therapy in Bulgaria. Medicina (Kaunas, Lithuania). 2019;**55**(7):pii:E313

[98] Pancholy S, Sharma P, Phancholy D, Patel T, Callans D, Marchlinski F. Meta-analysis of gender differences in residual stroke risk and major bleeding in patients with nonvalvular atrial fibrillation treated with oral anticoagulants. The American Journal of Cardiology. 2014;**113**:485-490

[99] Moseley A, Doukky R, Williams KA, Jaffer AK, Volgman AS. Indirect comparison of novel oral anticoagulants in women with nonvalvular atrial fibrillation. Journal of Women's Health (2002). 2017;**26**(3):214-221

[100] Reddy VY, Doshi SK, Kar S, Gibson DN, Price MJ, Huber K, et al. 5-year outcomes after left atrial appendage closure: From the PREVAIL and PROTECT AF trials. Journal of the American College of Cardiology. 2017;**70**(24):2964-2975

[101] Lee RJ, Lakkireddy D, Mittal S, Ellis C, Connor JT, Saville BR, et al. Percutaneous alternative to the maze procedure for the treatment of persistent or long-standing persistent atrial fibrillation (aMAZE trial): Rationale and design. American Heart Journal. 2015;**170**(6):1184-1194

Chapter 3

Anticoagulation in AF and Elderly Frail Patient: How to Face New Challenges

Alba María Costa Grille, Irene Criado Martín and Roberto Petidier Torregrossa

Abstract

Aging is an important risk factor for patients with atrial fibrillation. The estimated prevalence of atrial fibrillation in patients aged ≥80 years is 9–10%, with four- to fivefold increased risk of embolic stroke and with an estimated increased stroke risk of 1.45-fold per decade in aging. Older age is also associated with increased risk of major bleeding with oral anticoagulant (OAC) therapy. In this chapter, we will focus on the role of oral anticoagulation with new oral anticoagulants, non-vitamin K antagonist, in populations with common comorbid conditions, including age; chronic kidney disease; coronary artery disease, on multiple medication; and frailty. In patients 75 years and older, randomized trials have shown new oral anticoagulants to be as effective as warfarin, or in some cases superior, with an overall better safety profile, consistently reducing rates of intracranial hemorrhages. Prior to considering oral anticoagulant therapy in an elderly frail patient, a comprehensive assessment should be performed to include the risk and benefits, stroke risk, baseline kidney function, cognitive status, mobility and falling risk, multiple medication, nutritional status assessment, and life expectancy.

Keywords: anticoagulation, atrial fibrillation, elderly, new oral anticoagulants, frailty

1. Introduction

Atrial fibrillation (AF) is the most common arrhythmia in our daily clinical practice, affecting 4.5 million people in Europe and approximately 33.5 million people globally [1]. Estimates suggest a significant increase in AF incidence with age from 4.1/1000 under 75 years to 26.3/1000 in people older than 75 years [2]; in the same way, its prevalence rises from 0.1% in people under 55 years to 9% of those older than 80 [3–5], with an average annual cost of 2.365 € for each patient [6]. Due to the increase in life expectancy, the number of elderly people over 80 years with non-valvular AF (NVAF) will be fourfold in 2050; therefore, this group will represent over the 50% of the total of patients with this arrhythmia [4, 5], and stroke risk will increase 25–36% in elderly individuals between 80 and 89 years old [2, 7, 8].

Although people over 75 years present worse prognosis, higher mortality, and more adverse effects than those with age between 65 and 74 years [8], up to 35% of octogenarians do not receive oral anticoagulant (OAC) therapy [5]. The use of vitamin K antagonists (VKA) is reduced up to 14% for each decade of increase in age, regardless of other stroke risk factors [5, 9]. Frequent reasons for not initiating antithrombotic treatment in frail older individuals are (1) antiplatelet therapy, (2) more than 90 years, (3) falling risk, and (4) nursing home residents, even though a strong indication and evidence show that frailty increases stroke risk but not major bleeding risk [10].

In Europe, since 2011, there is an available new family of OAC with indication for stroke and venous thromboembolism prevention in patients with NVAF. This new family includes four direct oral anticoagulants (DOACs), dabigatran (an active direct thrombin inhibitor), apixaban, edoxaban, and rivaroxaban (direct factor Xa inhibitors). Different meta-analyses have proved up to 20% reduced stroke risk, 12% reduced mortality, and 50% reduced intracranial bleeding risk, in comparison with warfarin, showing fewer drugs and food interactions, with no control needed [9, 11]. The cost-utility of these drugs has been tested by cost-effectiveness analysis [6], and benefits shown are maintained regardless of age, presenting a greater reduction on all-cause mortality, stroke, and major, intracranial, and total bleedings in older individuals, the ones that present a higher risk [12–14].

Nonetheless, studies specifically designed in elderly population are not yet available, and the current evidence exclude multimorbidity patients, polypharmacy, and geriatric syndromes and just evaluate the benefit using health indicators with low clinical impact in this population [15–17]. In addition, the mean age of the patients included in clinical trials is 5–10 years lower than mean age of real-life patients with NVAF; because of that, the current guidelines are not able to make strong recommendations for individuals of 85 years or more [5, 18]. In order to solve this lack of evidence, data from sub-group phase III pivotal trials have been used, including over 30,000 patients older than 75 years, to demonstrate efficacy of DOACs in comparison to VKA, showing equal safety profile in the older ones than in younger people [9, 19, 20] (**Figure 1**).

Anticoagulation in elderly patients supposes a huge challenge because of the frequent association with health conditions that can modify not only the therapy indication but also the type and dosage of drug, tolerance, adhesion, safety profile, and the results we seek. Among these health determinants, we highlight frailty, disability, comorbidity, polypharmacy, cognitive impairment, risk of falling, nursing home residents, nutritional status, oral feeding problems, sensory disorder, and personal and social issues [2, 21]. A complete comprehensive geriatric assessment (CGA) focused in identifying all these factors, combined with aging biology knowledge, a good

	RE-LY4 Dabigatran	ROCKET5 Rivaroxaban	ARISTOTLE1 Apixaban	AVERROES2 Apixaban	ENGAGE3 Edoxaban
Total	18,113	14,264	18,201	5,599	21,105
≥75 years (%)	7,258 (40)	6,229 (44)	5,678 (31)	1,898 (34)	8,474 (40)
Old olders	≥85 a (4%) N=722	≥85 a (4.6%) N=663	≥80 a (13%) N=2,436 ≥90 a (0.5%) N=84	≥85 a (7%) N=366	≥85 a (4%)

1. Halvorsen S, et al. Eur Heart J 2014;35:1864–1872;
2. Ng KH, et al. Age Ageing 2016;45:73–77;
3. Giugliano RP, et al. New Engl J Med 2013;369:2093–2104 (Supplementary Appendix);
4. Eikelboom JW, et al. Circulation 2011;123:2363–2372;
5. Halperin JL, et al. Circulation 2014;130:138–146
6. Kato ET, et al. J Am Heart Assoc 2016; 5(5): e003432 DOI: 10.1161/JAHA.116.003432.

Figure 1.
Rates of very elderly subjects present in pivotal studies of DOAC.

calculation of global and disability-free life expectancy, and a better knowledge of elderly pharmacology and individuality side effects of OAC in this population including long time to benefit, will allow us to get a better adequacy of this therapy and to reach better health results. More clinical trials including frail aging patients and all these factors are needed in order to achieve real-life elderly population representative samples to better adjust OAC therapy in this group of age [18, 22].

2. Medication considerations in elderly patients

2.1 Thromboembolic and bleeding risk

The thrombotic risk in patients with NVAF is stratified by the CHA2DS2-VASc score: in patients with CHA2DS2-VASc score of 0, the thrombotic risk does not overweigh the risk of bleeding, so OAC is not recommended, but a CHA2DS2-VASc score of 1 or more reverses the risk/benefit balance, and anticoagulation is clearly recommended with class IA indication [23, 24].

The uncertainty arises when the score is 1; as in these patients, the stroke rate varies widely.

The thrombotic risk increase with higher CHA2DS2-VASc score. In elderly patients (75 years or older), OAC is always suitable; however, we may assess each case individually and evaluate bleeding risk, which is the most important complication in the anticoagulation treatment [24, 25].

Bleeding events are the most important complication of antithrombotic treatment, so this requires us to personalize decision-making, especially in elderly patients with multimorbidity, geriatric syndromes, frailty, or disability.

There are several scores that help us to measure bleeding risk [26], which take into account different factors associated with increasing bleeding risk, with no intention of contraindicating OAC but to modify them with our intervention, in order to increase anticoagulation therapy's security profile.

The most widespread one is HAS-BLED score, which includes different determinants, all of them potentially modifiable, except the age. Other scores, like HEMORR2HAGES score, add some aspects that are usually included in CGA (falls, cognitive impairment) susceptible to evaluation and management by a geriatrician. The ATRIA bleeding risk score takes into account five parameters and stratify the bleeding risk into three levels [27, 28]. The ORBIT risk score proposes five determinants: age, anemia, previous bleeding episodes, renal impairment, and antiplatelet therapy. This one demonstrates similar discrimination with better sizing than HAS-BLED and ATRIA scores, according to ROCKET AF trial [29]. The ABC-bleeding score includes age, previous bleeding episodes, and three serum biomarkers (hemoglobin, troponin T, and GDF15 or cystatin C/creatinine clearance) and obtains more appropriated results than HAS-BLED and the ORBIT, according to ARISTOTLE and RE-LY trials [27], but biomarkers are not standardized, and there is no defined cut point (class IIb indication).

2.2 Suitable control of anticoagulation

Antithrombotic treatment efficacy mostly depends on an adequate maintenance of anticoagulation levels, universally measured in VKA treatment by the "international normalized ratio" or INR (therapeutic range from 2.0 to 3.0).

The poor control of anticoagulation according to INR represents one of the independent predictors most related with thrombotic and bleeding complications showing in several trials [30].

Different methods have been proposed to define VKA anticoagulation quality like control percentage out of therapeutic range, control cross-sectional analysis, and time in therapeutic range (TRT), being the last one the most widely accepted and related with complication incidence (stroke, bleeding, and mortality) [30].

The INR is considered suboptimal when TRT calculated by Rosendaal method [31] (assumes a linear progression between two INR values and calculates the specific INR for each day) is fewer than 65%. Actually, labile INR is one of the items included in HAS-BLED score, and whereas an INR value above 70% is associated with an optimal efficacy and security level, lower values increase stroke risk, major bleeding, and mortality, associating even worse prognosis than patients with NVAF not receiving antithrombotic treatment.

2.3 Frailty and falls

Frail elderly patients with NVAF must be considerately able to receive anticoagulation therapy, because of their increased vulnerability and higher functional worsening risk and disability. It is necessary to properly distinguish in the differentiation between frailty (autonomous elderly with risk of functional impairment) and disability (functional impairment established with a greater or lesser degree of autonomy) of dependency (established disability). Frailty might precede by several years the development of disability and other clinical outcomes and is a major risk factor for non-catastrophic disability [32].

The comprehensive geriatric assessment (CGA) associated with performance status test, like short performance physical battery (SPPB) or gait speed measurement, is the suitable tool to assess an individualized therapeutic decision [33–35]. Once we identify a frailty elderly, we must initiate multicomponent exercise intervention that has demonstrated reduction of multimorbidity, disability, dependence, and, thus, institutionalization and death.

Oral anticoagulation has been proposed to increase intracranial bleeding risk due to traumatic brain injury related with falls, and this has been used as a contraindication to initiate anticoagulation, increasing its under prescription as the result [36]. The evidence is limited because patients with falls are excluded from trials and also there are papers that deny that patients with OAC and higher risk of falls have increased risk of severe bleedings [37].

However, the benefit in patients with high risk (CHA2DS2-VASc >3) exceeds the risk of falls [38]. It has been estimated that a patient with anticoagulation treatment has to fall 295 times in a year so that the risk exceeds benefit of treatment [39]. Between DOACs, only edoxaban was assessed in patients with atrial fibrillation judged to be at increased risk of falling. No treatment interaction was observed between either dosing regimens of edoxaban and warfarin for the efficacy and safety outcomes. Treatment with edoxaban resulted in a greater absolute risk reduction in severe bleeding events and all-cause mortality compared with warfarin [40].

2.4 Polypharmacy

Polypharmacy is defined as the chronic administration of five or more drugs, and this may determine OAC's choice, because risk of interactions is higher with a bigger number of medicines.

VKA treatments have frequent pharmacological interactions that require strict monitoring in disease exacerbating phases, treatment modifications, or hospital admission.

DOACs interact with fewer drugs and offer a more stable level of anticoagulation, being indicated in patients with polypharmacy. All of them are dependent on

P-glycoprotein (Pgp) transport for intestinal absorption. So concomitant use of inhibitors of this transport (amiodarone, ketoconazole, quinidine and verapamil) is expected to increase absorption and plasma concentration of DOACs, and inducers (rifampicin and carbamacepine) led to a decrease of its. Rivaroxaban and apixaban are partially metabolized by cytochrome P450 (CYP3A4), so agents considered inhibitors (azolic antifungals, ritonavir, and macrolides) increase the effect, and inducers (rifampicin, phenytoin, carbamazepine, and phenobarbital) reduce it [8, 41].

2.5 Nutritional status

Attention to nutrition is fundamental to good clinical practice. Nutrition care improves patient outcomes and reduces healthcare costs. The feed MEGlobal Group on Nutrition in Healthcare proposed Nutrition Care Pathway recommending the steps: screen always, intervene promptly when needed, and supervene routinely [42].

The nutritional status may affect OAC activity; thus, protein deficit and hypoalbuminemia in malnutrition patients raise plasma OAC concentration and, therefore, bleeding risk. Because of that, every elderly patient with NVAF may undergo nutritional status assessment before to initiate oral anticoagulation. As a screening tool, Mini Nutritional Assessment Short Form (MNA-SF) is the one recommended to identify malnutrition patients and the ones in risk for it [43].

2.6 Cognitive impairment

Dementia is not an anticoagulation contraindication by itself. Factors as severity, life expectancy, and adherence to therapy must be taken into account before indicating antithrombotic treatment [28].

Elderly patients with mild to moderate cognitive impairment ("Global Deterioration Scale" or GDS <5) have not increased bleeding risk and may receive OAC [2].

Labile INR in patients with VKA is related with progression of cognitive impairment; thus, we should consider to change DOACs in patients with moderate impair of cognitive function [8].

We do not know the bleeding risk or the benefit of anticoagulation therapy in patients with NVAF and severe cognitive impairment (GDS 6–7), but this phase of dementia is related with greater mortality and poor quality of life [33]. Therefore, not initiating OAC is an option if we reach an agreement with family/caregiver.

Cognitive impairment determines poor therapy adherence, so OAC should be initiated in patients with a responsible caregiver [2].

2.7 Mobility and disability

To evaluate the instrumental activities of daily life is useful to assess the independence to manage the medication, and to evaluate basic activities of daily life determines the access to INR control. These are two essential tools that may help to choose DOACs because they can improve adherence and security [2].

Although there is no evidence about OAC therapy risk/benefit ratio in patients with severe/total functional dependence, this situation is related with increase short- and long-term mortality and poor quality of life [30]; thus, it is fair to not indicate anticoagulation in these patients.

2.8 Life expectancy

The total life expectancy and free of disability may modify anticoagulation attitude in the elderly with NVAF. Currently, life expectancy varies a lot around the world from the higher one of 84.1 years in Japan to the lowest one of 52.2 years in Sierra Leone. Because of that, different tools have been designed and validated to assess life expectancy in order to take the right decision, not only based on age but also considering function, frailty, and comorbidity, among other factors. Some of the most used ones are Schonberg index and Lee index, both of them available in http://ePrognosis.ucsf.edu, and Studentski tables of life expectancy according to gait speed published in 2011 [44].

The time that an intervention takes until it shows efficacy (lag time to benefit) may be taken into account as well. Managing anticoagulation therapy, this time to benefit is really short, so life expectancy over 6 months is enough to justify anti-thrombotic drug use.

3. Dosage and profile of anticoagulant agent

Different meta-analyses [19, 20, 45, 46] have evaluated clinical randomized trials in patients over 75 years and have shown that DOACs are as effective in ictus prevention as warfarin; however, there are differences between type of OAC and dosage in the case of ictus/thromboembolism rate, major bleeding, and intracranial bleeding [47, 48]. Apixaban and edoxaban demonstrated less incidence of major bleeding in comparison with VKA; nevertheless, rivaroxaban and dabigatran 110 mg have similar risk. Apixaban, edoxaban, and dabigatran were associated with lower rates of intracranial bleeding compared to VKA [46].

Regarding gastrointestinal bleeding, in patients over 75 years, dabigatran and edoxaban 60 mg have demonstrated increased gastrointestinal bleeding risk in comparison with VKA, and there is no enough evidence in regard to apixaban and rivaroxaban [14, 45].

A recent review establishes that in patients older than 75 years, apixaban 5 mg twice a day is a first choice and rivaroxaban 20 mg once daily, edoxaban 60 mg once daily, and dabigatran 110 mg twice a day are second choices [49]. Given the increasing complexity of drug prescription in the elderly, in 2008 "Fit fOR The Aged (FORTA) classification" was born with intent to guide clinicians to optimize it. Recently, a systematic review of scientific evidence plus the application of Delphi method and FORTA classification has been published assessing oral anticoagulation in elderly patients with AF taking into account efficacy, security, and tolerability. Among DOACs, only apixaban was included in category A (very beneficial) because it shows superiority in every endpoint, including major and intracranial bleeding, ictus prevention, and mortality [50]. Furthermore, real-life anticoagulation [51–53] use trials have been published recently showing similar results to pivotal trials.

4. Special considerations for dosing in the elderly

There are no randomized clinical trials evaluating anticoagulation effectiveness and safety of the DOACs versus VKA in the clinical situations outlined below. The following recommendations are based on pivotal analyses of each of the new anticoagulants.

4.1 Elderly patient with renal failure

Chronic renal failure is a risk factor for both stroke and systemic embolism and in patients with atrial fibrillation (AF) [54]. Some studies using VKA have demonstrated the overall benefit of anticoagulation in patients with moderate to severe renal insufficiency (creatinine clearance 15–49 ml/min) despite the increased risk of bleeding [55].

In patients with mild to moderate renal failure, direct anticoagulants have been shown to decrease the incidence of systemic thromboembolism and major bleeding compared to VKA [56].

Regarding safety in patients with moderate renal insufficiency (CrCl 30–49 ml/min), apixaban has been shown to significantly reduce the risk of bleeding against VKA. No significant differences were found between dabigatran and rivaroxaban versus VKA [57]. Severe renal failure (CrCl <30 ml/min) was an exclusion criterion in the pivotal clinical trials of DOACs.

Analyzing pharmacokinetic properties, it is important to point out that 80% of dabigatran is eliminated by the kidneys, while in the case of rivaroxaban, apixaban, and edoxaban, the renal clearance is 35, 25, and 50, respectively. Based on this, dabigatran is contraindicated in patients with CrCl<30 ml/min and all "anti-factor X" when the CrCl is less than 15 ml/min [15].

In patients with severe renal failure (CrCl <15 ml/min), including dialysis patients, clinical guidelines suggest not to anticoagulate [15].

4.2 Elderly patient with liver failure

Metabolism through cytochrome P450 (CYP3A4) is null or insignificant in dabigatran and edoxaban, about 25% in apixaban and 30% in rivaroxaban.

In mild hepatic insufficiency with no alteration of coagulation, the use of DOACs is safe, although it is recommended to avoid concomitant use with other drugs that are metabolized by CYP or glycoprotein P [58]. Moderate to severe hepatic failure (Child-Pugh B or C) is a contraindication for anticoagulation with both VKA and DOACs.

4.3 Elderly patient with malnutrition or dysphagia

Unlike VKA, DOACs do not interact with elements of the diet. Data available for elderly people with low weight and corporal mass index are poor. Current recommendations subscribe not to modify the doses of rivaroxaban or dabigatran in patients with low weight. In patients with <60 kg, the dose of edoxaban should be set (30 mg/24 h) and is one of the two criteria necessary to recommend the dose reduction of apixaban (2.5 mg/12 h) [48].

The DOAC binding-protein coefficient is variable: 35% dabigatran, 50% edoxaban, 90% apixaban, and > 90% rivaroxaban [58]. There are no specific recommendations in this regard, and the published data do not indicate to modify the doses [15].

4.4 Elderly patient with a history of bleeding

In elderly patients with an episode of major bleeding, whether intracranial or digestive, in treatment with anticoagulants, it is recommended to individualize the decision of restarting anticoagulation, based on several conditions such as age, control of blood pressure, the origin of bleeding, suitable anticoagulation at the time of the bleeding, the need for antiplatelet therapy, the risk of ischemic stroke, and, in the case of intracranial origin, the location and severity of it. Anticoagulation should be initiated after treatment of the cause, with anticoagulants with a low risk of bleeding, waiting 4–8 weeks if the origin was intracranial [49].

4.5 Elderly patient with cancer or terminal organ disease

There is no available evidence to establish recommendations on anticoagulant therapy in elderly patients with atrial fibrillation and cancer or terminal organ disease. In cancer patients with atrial fibrillation, the low efficacy and safety of VKA have been documented given the interactions with cancer treatment [55]. In this scenario, DOACs could provide great advantages due to their predictable action at fixed doses. Possible limitations would come from the hemorrhagic risk, especially in gastrointestinal and central nervous system tumors, and the potential interactions with antineoplastic treatment, especially if metabolized via CYP or glycoprotein P. In the case of terminal organ disease, the prescription of drugs that prolong life or prevent disability should be avoided or interrupted, especially if the time necessary to obtain the benefit exceeds life expectancy. With regard to anticoagulants, it is recommended to suspend whenever the life expectancy is less than 6 months and is not a case of high thromboembolic risk [2, 59, 60].

4.6 Elderly patient during the perioperative period and surgery

DOACs, unlike VKA, can be maintained perioperatively, without the need for bridging therapy with heparin, given that their half-life is short, and the anticoagulant effect decreases rapidly after stopping the drug. Taking into account renal function and the risk of bleeding from surgery, a safety time period prior to the intervention can be established without the need for biological control [61].

In invasive procedures with low or moderate risk of bleeding, the anti-factor Xa must be suspended 24 hours before the intervention and 36 hours, in the event of severe renal insufficiency (CrCl <30 ml/min). In the case of dabigatran, the withdrawal should be 24–48 hours before, depending on the glomerular filtration rate. In high-risk bleeding procedures, anti-factor Xa must be discontinued 48 hours before the intervention and dabigatran 48–96 hours according to the glomerular filtration rate.

If urgent intervention is required, the procedure should be delayed at least the half-life of the drug (approximately 12 hours average) provided there is an end of effect parallel to the half-life (dabigatran, apixaban, and edoxaban) and considering the degree of renal elimination (25% apixaban, 50% edoxaban, and 80% dabigatran).

If this is not possible, there is an increased risk of bleeding that must be assessed against the urgency of the intervention. Prothrombin complex concentrates or recombinant factor VIIa should be used only in the event of significant hemorrhage, and not for prophylactic reversal [62]. In 2015, the European Medicine Agency approved the use of idarucizumab, a humanized monoclonal antibody, to reverse the effects of dabigatran in life-threatening bleeding episodes. Although not yet commercialized in Europe [63], the use of andexanet alfa has been tested for the reversal of the effects of the factor Xa inhibitors with favorable and promising results in elderly patients, still awaiting approval [64].

The resumption of treatment will depend on the postoperative hemorrhagic risk. In the case of major or urological abdominal surgery, we should wait for the absence of active hemorrhage visualized by the drainages. In procedures with good hemostasis, it can be restarted 6 hours after the intervention, but normally the indications are to restart anticoagulation 24 hours after the intervention; unless there is a high risk of bleeding, then it is suitable to wait 48/72 hours [65].

In dental extractions and other dental procedures, there is currently no knowledge enough to establish recommendations with a high level of evidence. In the bibliography, being a low-risk procedure, it recommends limiting the extractions to a maximum of two or three pieces and not stopping the anticoagulant treatment. It is recommended to perform the intervention about 12 hours after the last dose and not to take the next dose of DOAC until a good hemostasis is achieved, around 6 hours later [66].

4.7 Nonagenarian and centennial patients

There are no data available on the efficacy and safety of DOACs in nonagenarian and centennial patients [67]. As age increases, the risk of atrial fibrillation and embolism increases but also of bleeding [68]. Apixaban is the DOAC that has less renal elimination, and, compared to the VKA, apixaban and edoxaban at low doses (30 mg) are those that had lower rates of major hemorrhages in this age group, although the latter was less effective in the prevention of ischemic stroke. A subanalysis of the ARISTOTLE study concludes that patients with atrial fibrillation and a single associated factor (advanced age, low body weight, or renal dysfunction) have an increased risk of stroke or systemic embolism and major bleeding but show consistent benefits with the dose of 5 mg twice daily of apixaban vs. warfarin compared to patients without these characteristics. The dose of apixaban 5 mg twice daily is safe, effective, and appropriate for patients with only one dose-reduction criterion [69]. There is a study that indicates that there is an increased risk of ischemic stroke or systemic embolic event, in patients with a dose of apixaban 2.5 versus warfarin [70].

4.8 Elderly patient with poor therapeutic compliance or social isolation

The lack of adherence to chronic treatment with oral anticoagulants increases the risk of thromboembolic and hemorrhagic complications [71]. Multiple reasons have been described associated with the lack of adherence to anticoagulant treatment in the elderly, such as neuropsychiatric pathology, social situation, or lack of understanding of the disease [72]. DOACs present the advantages of the fixed dosage and do not need monitoring, which could improve the adherence and persistence of the treatment [71, 73, 74].

However, the transition from VKA to DOAC has not always been shown to ensure therapeutic compliance, which is even more important since this pharmacological group has a shorter half-life than VKA [22]. Therefore, an analysis of the reasons for nonadherence should always be performed before taking the anticoagulation decision and choosing the type of anticoagulant [1–31, 33–39, 43–69, 75–77] as well as, if indicated, carrying out strategies to ensure compliance with long-term treatment, regardless of the type of anticoagulant [78].

It is known that therapeutic regimens of a single dose per day can improve adherence [79], although this aspect is questioned given the variability of drug concentration and the risk of events when a dose is forgotten [80].

5. Comprehensive geriatric assessment before making a decision about OAC

As a result of what was previously exposed, it has been proposed to carry out a complete comprehensive geriatric assessment before to initiate anticoagulation treatment in people over 75 years with NVAF. The first step would be to assess a Barthel Index and Reisberg's GDS scale as represented in **Figure 2** [75]. Apart from the presence of Barthel Index ≥85 or GDS scale ≤5, it is also recommended to assess the short physical performance battery (SPPB) to identify frailty [35]. If frailty condition

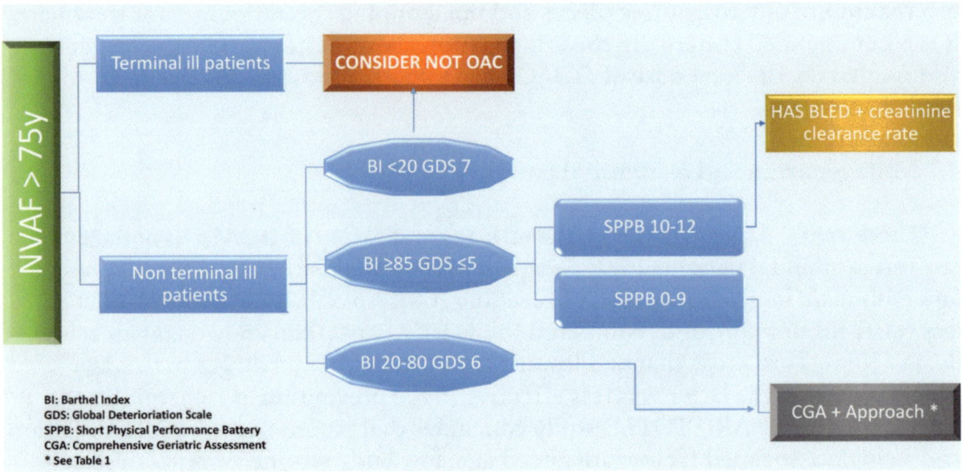

Figure 2.
Algorithm deciding oral anticoagulation in older patients. Modified from Petidier et al. [75].

CGA	Approach
CIRS-G	Prioritization
MNA-SF	Nutritional supplementation
Falls	Falling risk factor assessment Multicomponent exercise
Polypharmacy	STOPP/START

Table 1.
Comprehensive geriatric assessment and possible approaches before OAC.

was detected, Barthel Index is between 25 and 80, or if GDS scale is 6, it is necessary to include a comprehensive geriatric assessment with a Mini Nutritional Assessment Short Form (MNA-SF®) [43] for nutritional status, CIRS-G scale [76] to evaluate comorbidity], and STOPP/START criteria [77] to assess falling risk and polypharmacy and to identify potentially inappropriate medicines. Personalized anticoagulation use is the most important approach (**Table 1**).

6. Summary box

- The selection of the anticoagulant drug and its dose should be carried out individually and carefully, taking into account clinical, geriatric criteria, and the preferences of the patient.

- It seems reasonable that patients who do not receive such treatment should be limited to those with an obvious contraindication and those who are considered in short value because they are in the last days of their lives with very high competitive risks.

- In patients >75 years old, DOACs as a class were superior to warfarin with respect to both efficacy and safety, showing similar efficacy in the prevention of stroke and systemic embolization between them but with lowest risk of major bleeding for apixaban and lower rates of intracranial hemorrhage for apixaban, edoxaban, and dabigatran (than rivaroxaban or warfarin).

Conflict of interest

Alba María Costa Grille and Irene Criado Martín declare no conflict of interest. Roberto Petidier Torregrossa is a consultant for Bristol-Myers Squibb Company/ Pfizer Inc. and Daiichi Sankyo.

Author details

Alba María Costa Grille, Irene Criado Martín and Roberto Petidier Torregrossa*
Geriatrics Department, University Hospital of Getafe, Madrid, Spain

*Address all correspondence to: roberto.petidier@salud.madrid.org

References

[1] Chugh SS, Haymoeller R, Narayanan K, Singh D, Rienstra M, Benjamin EJ, et al. Worldwide epidemiology of atrial fibrillation: A global burden of disease 2010 study. Circulation. 2014;**129**:837-847

[2] Granziera S, Cohen AT, Nante G, Manzato E, Sergi G. Thromboembolic prevention in frail elderly patients with atrial fibrillation: A practical algorithm. Journal of the American Medical Directors Association. 2015;**16**:358-364

[3] Guindo Soldevila J, Martínez Ruíz MD, Duran Robert I, Tornos P, Martínez-Rubio A. Evaluación de riesgo tromboembólico y hemorrágico de los pacientes con fibrilación auricular. Revista Española de Cardiología Suplementos. 2013;**13**:9-13

[4] Go AS, Hylek EM, Phillips KA, Chang Y, Henault LE, Selby JV, et al. Prevalence of diagnosed atrial fibrillation in adults national implications for rhythm management and stroke prevention: The anticoagulation and risk factors In atrial fibrillation (ATRIA) study. JAMA. 2001;**285**:2370-2375

[5] Lefebvre MC, St-Onge M, Glazer-Cavanagh M, Bell L, Kha Nguyen JN, Viet-Quoc Nguyen P, et al. The effect of bleeding risk and frailty status on anticoagulation patterns in octogenarians with atrial fibrillation: The FRAIL-AF study. The Canadian Journal of Cardiology. 2016;**32**:169-176

[6] Barón Esquivias G, Escolar Albadalejo G, Zamorano JL, Betegón Nicolás L, Canal Fontcuberta C, Salas-Cansado M, et al. Análisis coste-efectividad de apixabán frente a acenocumarol en la prevención del ictus en pacientes con fibrilación auricular no valvular en España. Revista Española de Cardiología. 2015;**68**:680-690

[7] Annoni G, Mazzola P. Real-world characteristics of hospitalized frail elderly patients with atrial fibrillation: Can we improve the current prescription of anticoagulants? Journal of Geriatric Cardiology. 2016;**13**:226-232

[8] Suárez Fernández C, Formiga F, Camafort M, Cepeda Rodrigo M, Díez-Manglano J, Pose Reino A, et al. Antithrombotic treatment in elderly patients with atrial fibrillation: A practical approach. BMC Cardiovascular Disorders. 2015;**15**:143

[9] Edholm K, Ragle N, Rondina MT. Antihrombotic management of atrial fibrillation in the elderly. The Medical Clinics of North America. 2015;**99**:417-430

[10] Maes F, Dalleur O, Henrard S, Wouters D, Scavée C, Spinewine A, et al. Risk scores and geriatric profile: Can they really help us in anticoagulation decision making among older patients suffering from atrial fibrillation? Clinical Interventions in Aging. 2014;**9**:1091-1099

[11] De Caterina R, Husted S, Wallentin L, Andreotti F, Arnesen H, Bachmann F, et al. New oral anticoagulants in atrial fibrillation and acute coronary syndromes. Journal of the American College of Cardiology. 2012;**59**:1413-1425

[12] Halvorsen S, Atar D, Yang H, De Caterina R, Erol C, Garcia D, et al. Efficacy and safety of apixaban compared with warfarin according to age for stroke prevention in atrial fibrillation: Observations from the ARISTOTLE trial. European Heart Journal. 2014;**35**:1864-1872

[13] Halperin JL, Hankey GJ, Wojdyla DM, Piccini JP, Lokhnygina Y, Patel MR, et al. Efficacy and safety of rivaroxaban compared with

warfarin among elderly patients with nonvalvular atrial fibrillation in the rivaroxaban once daily, Oral, direct factor Xa inhibition compared with vitamin K antagonism for prevention of stroke and embolism trial in atrial fibrillation (ROCKET AF). Circulation. 2014;**130**:138-146

[14] Kato ET, Giugliano RP, Ruff CT, Koretsune Y, Yamashita T, Kiss RG, et al. Efficacy and safety of edoxaban in elderly patients with atrial fibrillation in the ENGAGE AF-TIMI 48 trial. Journal of the American Heart Association. 2016;**5**:e003432. DOI: 10.1161/JAHA.116.003432

[15] Kirchhof P, Benussi S, Kotecha D, Ahlsson A, Atar D, Casadei M, et al. ESC guidelines for the management of atrial fibrillation developed in collaboration with EACTS. The task force for the management of atrial fibrillation of the European Society of Cardiology (ESC). European Heart Journal. 2016;**37**:2893-2962

[16] Heidenreich PA, Solis P, Estes NAM 3rd, Fonarow GC, Jurgens CY, Marine JE, et al. 2016 ACC/AHA clinical performance and quality measures for adults with atrial fibrillation or atrial flutter: A report of the American College of Cardiology/American Heart Association task force on performance measures. Journal of the American College of Cardiology. 2016;**68**:525-568

[17] Senoo K, Lau YC, Lip GY. Updated Nice guideline. Management of Atrial fibrillation. Expert Review of Cardiovascular Therapy. 2014;**12**:1037-1040

[18] Rich MW, Chyun DA, Skolnick AH, Alexander KP, Forman DE, Kitzman DW, et al. Knowledge gaps in cardiovascular care of the older adult population: A scientific statement from the American Heart Association, American College of Cardiology, and American Geriatrics Society. Journal of the American College of Cardiology. 2016;**67**:2419-2440

[19] Sardar P, Chatterjee S, Chaudhari S, Lip GY. New oral anticoagulants in elderly adults: Evidence from a meta-analysis of randomized trials. Journal of the American Geriatrics Society. 2014;**62**:857-864

[20] Bai Y, Guo S-D, Deng H, Shantsila A, Fauchier L. Effectiveness and safety of oral anticoagulants in older patients with atrial fibrillation: A systematic review and meta-regression analysis. Age and Ageing. 2017:1-9

[21] Sennesael AL, Dogné JM, Spinewine A. Optimizing the safe use of direct oral anticoagulants in older patients: A teachable moment. JAMA Internal Medicine. 2015;**175**:1608-1609

[22] Wuthzler A, Ulmenstein S, Attanasio P, Huemer M, Shoker A, Hendrik L, et al. Treatment of nonagenarians with atrial fibrillation: Insights from the Berlin atrial Fibrillation (BAF) registry. Journal of the American Medical Directors Association. 2015;**16**:969-972

[23] Denoël P, Vanderstraeten J, Mols P, Pepersack T. Could some geriatric characteristics hinder the prescription of anticoagulants in atrial fibrillation in the elderly? Journal of Aging Research. 2014;**2014**:693740. DOI: 10.1155/2014/603740 Epub 2014 Sep 10

[24] Veiga F, Malfeito MR, Barros SM, Magariños MM. La anticoagulación oral en el anciano con fibrilación auricular no valvular. Revista Española de Geriatría y Gerontología. 2015;**50**:134-142

[25] Gil P. Reflexiones en torno a la anticoagulación en el anciano. Medicina Clínica (Barcelona). 2016;**147**:151-153

[26] Thomas IC, Sorrentino MJ. Bleeding risk prediction models in atrial

fibrillation. Current Cardiology Reports. 2014;**16**:432

[27] Hijazi Z, Oldgren J, Lindbäck J, Alexander JH, Connolly SJ, Eikelboom JW, et al. The novel biomarker-based ABC (age, biomarkers, clinical history)-bleeding risk score for patients with atrial fibrillation: A derivation and validation study. Lancet. 2016;**387**:2302-2311

[28] Tavassoli N, Perrin A, Bérard E, Gillette S, Vellas B, Rolland Y, et al. Factors associated with undertreatment of atrial fibrillation in geriatric outpatients with Alzheimer disease. American Journal of Cardiovascular Drugs. 2013;**13**:425-433

[29] O'Brien EC, Simon DN, Thomas LE, Hylek EM, Gersh B, Ansell JE, et al. The ORBIT bleeding score: A simple bedside score to assess bleeding risk in atrial fibrillation. European Heart Journal. 2015;**36**:3258-3264

[30] Anguita Sánchez M, Beromeu Fernandez V, Cequier Fillat A. Quality of vitamin K antagonist anticoagulation in Spain: Prevalence of poor control and associated factors. Revista Española de Cardiología. 2015;**68**:761-768

[31] Rosendaal FR, Cannegieter SC, van der Meer FJ, Briet E. A method to determine the optimal intensity of oral anticoagulant therapy. Thrombosis and Haemostasis. 1993;**69**:236-239

[32] Rodriguez-Mañas L, Fried LP. Frailty in the clinical scenario. Lancet. 2015;**385**(9968):e7-e9

[33] Formiga F, Robles J, Fort I. Dementia, a progressive disease: Severe dementia. Identification of end-stage dementia. Revista Española de Geriatría y Gerontología. 2009;**44**:2-8

[34] Stineman MG, Xie D, Pan Q, Kurichi JE, Zhang Z, Saliba D, et al. All-cause 1-, 5-, and 10-year mortality in elderly people according to activities of daily living stage. Journal of the American Geriatrics Society. 2012;**60**:485-492

[35] Freiberger E, de Vreede P, Schoene D, Rydwik E, Mueller V, Frändin K, et al. Performance-based physical function in older community-dwelling persons. A systematic review of instruments. Age and Ageing. 2012;**41**:712-721

[36] Pugh D, Pugh J, Mead GE. Attitudes of physicians regarding anticoagulation for atrial fibrillation: A systematic review. Age and Ageing. 2011;**40**:675-683

[37] Donzé J, Clair C, Hug B, Rodondi N, Waeber G, Cornuz J, et al. Risk of falls and major bleeds in patients on oral anticoagulation therapy. The American Journal of Medicine. 2012;**125**:773-778

[38] Gage BF, Birman-Deych E, Kerzner R, Radford MJ, Nilasena DS, Rich MW. Incidence of intracranial hemorrhage in patients with atrial fibrillation who are prone to fall. The American Journal of Medicine. 2005;**118**:612-617

[39] Man-Son-Hing M, Nichol G, Lau A, Lauoacis A. Choosing antithrombotic therapy for elderly patients with atrial fibrillation who are at risk for falls. Archives of Internal Medicine. 1999;**159**:677-685

[40] Steffel J, Giugluano RP, Braunwald E, Murphy SA, Mercuri M, Choi Y, et al. Edoxaban versus warfarin in atrial fibrillation patients at risk of falling. ENGAGE AF–TIMI 48 analysis. Journal of the American College of Cardiology. 2016;**68**:1169-1178

[41] Verheugt FW, Granger CB. Oral anticoagulants for stroke prevention in atrial fibrillation: Current status, special situations, and unmet needs. Lancet. 2015;**386**:303-310

[42] Correia MI, Hegazi RA, Higashiguchi T, Michel JP, Reddy BR, Tappenden KA, et al. Evidence-based recommendations for addressing malnutrition in health care: An updated strategy from the feed M.E. global study group. Journal of the American Medical Directors Association. 2014;**15**:544-550

[43] Kaiser MJ, Bauer JM, Ramsch C, Uter W, Guigoz Y, Cederholm T, et al. Validation of the mini nutritional assessment short-form (MNA®-SF): A practical tool for identification of nutritional status. The Journal of Nutrition, Health & Aging. 2009;**13**:782-788

[44] Studenski S, Perera S, Patel K, Rosano C, Faulkner K, Inzitari M, et al. Gait speed and survival in older adults. JAMA. 2011;**305**:50-81

[45] Sharma M, Cornelius VR, Patel JP, Davies JG, Molokhia M. Efficacy and harms of direct oral anticoagulants in the elderly for stroke prevention in atrial fibrillation and secondary prevention of venous thromboembolism: Systematic review and meta-analysis. Circulation. 2015;**132**:194-204

[46] Malik AH, Yandrapalli S, Aronow WS, Panza JA, Cooper HA. Meta-analysis of direct-acting ora anticoagulants compared with warfarin in patients >75 years of age. The American Journal of Cardiology. 2019;**123**:2051-2057

[47] Capranzano P, Miccichè E, D'Urso L, Privitera F, Tamburino C. Personalizing oral anticoagulant treatment in patients with atrial fibrillation. Expert Review of Cardiovascular Therapy. 2013;**11**:959-973

[48] Turagam MK, Velagapudi P, Flaker GC. Stroke prevention in the elderly atrial fibrillation patient with comorbid conditions: Focus on non-vitamin K antagonist oral anticoagulants. Clinical Interventions in Aging. 2015;**10**:1431-1444

[49] Diener HC, Aisenberg J, Ansell J, Atar D, Breithardt G, Eikelboom J, et al. Choosing a particular oral anticoagulant and dose for stroke prevention in individual patients with non-valvular atrial fibrillation: Part 2. European Heart Journal. 2017;**38**:860-868

[50] Wehling M, Collins R, Gil VM, Hanon O, Hardt R, Hoffmeister M, et al. Appropriateness of oral anticoagulants for the long-term treatment of atrial fibrillation in older people: Results of an evidence-based review and international consensus validation process (OAC-FORTA 2016). Drugs & Aging. 2017;**34**:499-507

[51] Yao X, Abraham NS, Sangaralingham LR, Bellolio F, McBane RD, Shah ND, et al. Effectiveness and safety of dabigatran, rivaroxaban and apixaban versus warfarin in nonvalvular atrial fibrillation. Journal of the American Heart Association. 2016;**5**:e003725. DOI: 10.1161/JAHA.116.003725

[52] Noseworthy PA, Yao X, Abraham NS, Sangaralingham LR, McBane RD, Shah ND. Direct comparison of dabigatran, rivaroxaban and apixaban for effectiveness and safety in nonvalvular atrial fibrillation. Chest. 2016;**150**:1302-1312

[53] Vinogradova Y, Coupland C, Hill T, Hippisley-Cox J. Risks and benefits of dierct oral anticoagulants versus warfarin in a real world setting: Cohort study in primary care. BMJ. 2018;**362**:k2505

[54] Olesen JB, Lip GY, Kamper AL, Hommel K, Kober L, Lane DA, et al. Stroke and bleeding in atrial fibrillation with chronic kidney disease. The New England Journal of Medicine. 2012;**367**:625-635

[55] Friberg L, Benson L, Lip GY. Balancing stroke and bleeding risks in patients with atrial fibrillation and renal

failure: The Swedish atrial fibrillation cohort study. European Heart Journal. 2015;**36**:297-306

[56] Del-Carpio Munoz F, Gharacholou SM, Munger TM, Friedman PA, Asirvatham SJ, Packer DL, et al. Meta-analysis of renal function on the safety and efficacy of novel oral anticoagulants for atrial fibrillation. The American Journal of Cardiology. 2016;**117**:69-75

[57] Harel Z, Sholzberg M, Shah PS, Pavenski K, Harel S, Wald R, et al. Comparisons between novel oral anticoagulants and vitamin K antagonists in patients with CKD. JASN. 2014;**25**:431-442

[58] Rosanio S, Keylani AM, D'Agostino DC, DeLaughter CM, Vitarelli A. Pharmacology, benefits, unaddressed questions, and pragmatic issues of the newer oral anticoagulants for stroke prophylaxis in non-valvular atrial fibrillation and proposal of a management algorithm. International Journal of Cardiology. 2014;**174**:471-483

[59] O'Mahony D, O'Connor MN. Pharmacotherapy at the end-of-life. Age and Ageing. 2011;**40**:419-422

[60] Cruz-Jentoft AJ, Boland B, Rexach L. Drug therapy optimization at the end of life. Drugs & Aging. 2012;**29**:511-521

[61] Heidbuchel H, Verhamme P, Alings M, Antz M, Hacke W, Oldgren J, et al. European heart rhythm association practical guide on the use of new oral anticoagulants in patients with nonvalvular atrial fibrillation. EHRA Practical Guide. Europace. 2015;**17**:1467-1507. DOI: 10.1093/europace/euv309

[62] Niessner A, Tamargo J, Morais J, Koller L, Wassmann S, Husted SE, et al. Reversal strategies for non-vitamin K antagonist oral anticoagulants: A critical appraisal of available evidence and recommendations for clinical management—a joint position paper of the European Society of Cardiology Working Group on Cardiovascular Pharmacotherapy and European Society of Cardiology Working Group on Thrombosis. European Heart Journal. 2017;**38**:1710-1716

[63] Finks SW, Rogers KC. Idarucizumab (Praxbind®): The first reversal agent for a direct oral anticoagulant. The American Journal of Medicine. 2016. DOI: 10.1016/j.amjmed.2016.11.029. [Epub ahead of print]

[64] Connolly SJ, Milling TJ Jr, Eikelboom JW, Gibson CM, Curnutte JT, Gold A, et al. Andexanet alfa for acute major bleeding associated with factor Xa inhibitors. The New England Journal of Medicine. 2016;**375**:1131-1141

[65] Vivas D, Roldán I, Ferrandis R, Marín F, Roldán V, Tello-Montoliu A, et al. Manejoperioperatorioyperiprocedimiento del tratamiento antitrombótico: documento de consenso de SEC, SEDAR, SEACV, SECTCV, AEC, SECPRE, SEPD, SEGO, SEHH, SETH, SEMERGEN, SEMFYC, SEMG, SEMICYUC, SEMI, SEMES, SEPAR, SENEC, SEO, SEPA, SERVEI, SECOT y AEU. Revista Española de Cardiología. 2018;**71**:553-564. DOI: 10.1016/j.recesp.2018.01.001

[66] Altirriba J, Aparicio P. Anticoagulación oral en Atención Primaria. Revista Española de Sanidad Penitenciaria. 2017;**19**:28-44

[67] Stöllberger C, Brooks R, Finsterer J, Pachofszky T. Use of direct-acting oral anticoagulants in nonagenarians: A call for more data. Drugs & Aging. 2016;**33**:315-320

[68] Lip GY, Clementy N, Pericart L, Banerjee A, Fauchier L. Stroke and major bleeding risk in elderly patients aged ≥75 years with atrial fibrillation:

The Loire Valley atrial fibrillation project. Stroke. 2015;**46**:143-150

[69] Alexander JH et al. Apixaban 5 mg twice daily and clinical outcomes in patients with atrial fibrillation and advanced age, low body weight, or high creatinine a secondary analysis of a randomized clinical trial. JAMA Cardiology. 2016;**1**:673-681. DOI: 10.1001/jamacardio.2016.1829

[70] Nielsen PB, Skjøth F, Søgaard M, Kjældgaard JN, Lip GY, Larsen TB. Effectiveness and safety of reduced dose non-vitamin K antagonist oral anticoagulants and warfarin in patients with atrial fibrillation: Propensity weighted nationwide cohort study. British Medical Journal. 2017;**356**:j510

[71] Potpara TS, Lane DA, Lip GY. Optimizing stroke prevention in atrial fibrillation: Better adherence and compliance from patients and physicians leads to better outcomes. Europace. 2015;**17**:507-508

[72] Kneeland PP, Fang MC. Current issues in patient adherence and persistence: Focus on anticoagulants for the treatment and prevention of thromboembolism. Patient Preference and Adherence. 2010;**4**:51-60

[73] Zalesak M, Siu K, Francis K, Yu C, Alvrtsyan H, Rao Y, et al. Higher persistence in newly diagnosed nonvalvular atrial fibrillation patients treated with dabigatran versus warfarin. Circulation. Cardiovascular Quality and Outcomes. 2013;**6**:567-574

[74] Laliberte F, Cloutier M, Nelson WW, Coleman CI, Pilon D, Olson WH, et al. Real-world comparative effectiveness and safety of rivaroxaban and warfarin in nonvalvular atrial fibrillation patients. Current Medical Research and Opinion. 2014;**30**:1317-1325

[75] Petidier R, Abiazanda P, Nogueron A, Gonzalo M, Gutierrez J, Gil P, et al. Revista Española de Geriatría y Gerontología. 2018;**53**:344-355

[76] Miller MD, Paradis CF, Houck PR, Mazumdar S, Stack JA, et al. Rating chronic medical illness burden in geropsychiatric practice and research: Application of the Cumulative illness rating scale. Psychiatry Research. 1992;**41**:237-248

[77] O'Mahony D, O'Sullivan D, Byrne S, O'Connor MN, Ryan C, Gallagher P. STOPP/START criteria for potentially inappropriate prescribing in older people: Version 2. Age and Ageing. 2015;**44**:213-218

[78] Rodriguez RA, Carrier M, Wells PS. Non-adherence to new oral anticoagulants: A reason for concern during long-term anticoagulation? Journal of Thrombosis and Haemostasis. 2013;**11**:390-394

[79] Srivastava K, Arora A, Kataria A, Cappelleri JC, Sadosky A, Peterson AM. Impact of reducing dosing frequency on adherence to oral therapies: A literature review and meta-analysis. Patient Preference and Adherence. 2013;**7**:419-434

[80] Vrijens B, Heidbuchel H. Non-vitamin K antagonist oral anticoagulants: Considerations on once- vs. twice-daily regimens and their potential impact on medication adherence. Europace. 2015;**17**:514-523

Chapter 4

Antiarrhythmic Drugs in Atrial Fibrillation

Stefan Simović, Ivan Srejović, Vladimir Živković, Slobodanka Mitrović, Jovana Jeremić, Vladimir Jakovljević and Goran Davidović

Abstract

Atrial fibrillation (AF) represents the most common sustained heart rhythm abnormality. It presents in paroxysmal and persistent forms. The pathogenesis of AF is still debatable with several proposed mechanisms. The main pathway for diagnosis of AF is through electrocardiographic record. Treatment strategies can be divided into two strategies: rate and rhythm control. For rhythm control, antiarrhythmic drugs, direct current cardioversion, and electrophysiological ablation are used, while for rate control, chronotropic drugs are being used, while AV node ablation is required in order to reduce rapid ventricular rate, which is often observed in patients with AF. The rhythm control strategy implies the use of cardioversion to convert AF to normal, sinus rhythm. Cardioversion can be either pharmacological or electrical. Rate control strategy can be implied to patients with permanent AF but should also imply for the patients with paroxysmal AF when relapse occurs. Rapid ventricular rates can cause palpitations or even a syncope and other rate-related symptoms; however, these high ventricular rates lead to degradation of left ventricle performance, mitral regurgitation, and further dilatation of the left atrium. The main antiarrhythmic drugs used in treatment of AF are propafenone, flecainide, beta-blockers, amiodarone, dronedarone, dofetilide, vernakalant, and ranolazine.

Keywords: atrial fibrillation, antiarrhythmic drugs, propafenone, flecainide, amiodarone, dronedarone, dofetilide

1. Introduction

Atrial fibrillation (AF) represents the most common sustained heart rhythm abnormality, one of the most common cardiovascular diseases and a major cause of stroke in developed countries. It presents in paroxysmal and persistent forms. Paroxysmal form of AF is defined with a duration less than 7 days and can terminate spontaneously, while persistent forms are further classified as persistent and permanent forms with a duration of greater than 7 days with only difference in possibility of conversion to normal, sinus rhythm; in persistent form conversion to sinus rhythm is possible, while in permanent form, conversion to normal rhythm is not possible.

Atrial fibrillation can occur in isolated form (without associated comorbidities), yet it is more commonly seen with other cardiovascular diseases, cardiomyopathies, hypertension, diabetes mellitus, and obesity. When seen in association with these comorbidities, atrial fibrillation deeply affects quality of life and increases mortality and morbidity [1].

AF affects 1–1.5% of the population in the developed world with approximately 3 million people with a diagnosis of AF in the USA [2]. The prevalence and incidence of AF are sharply increased with age with a rise from 0.7% in the age group of 55–59 years to 17.8% in those aged 85 years or above. With such a big prevalence, treatment of AF represents a significant burden to the healthcare systems. The data from the US databases from 2001 showed the estimated total annual cost of AF treatment at 6.65 billion US$ [3].

The pathogenesis of AF is still debatable with several proposed mechanisms. The traditional theory suggests multiple reentrant atrial activation by migrating wavelets and contraction rate of 350–900 beats per minute [4, 5]. Several animal models have shown that AF is triggered by a focal source, which rapidly fires signals and is usually found in superior pulmonary veins. It stimulates multiple wavelet reentry mechanism within the atrial substrate or engages a spiral or rotor for the reentry [6–8]. Research also showed that in patients with AF, there is a sympathetic predominance over parasympathetic; however, in certain patients, it can be characterized with predominance of vagal or an adrenergic form of AF [9]. Besides that, AF can be related to temporary causes, such as drugs, alcohol, thyrotoxicosis, surgery, myocardial infarction, myocarditis, pericarditis, pulmonary embolism, and others. Obesity, sleep apnea and metabolic syndrome have also been linked to AF. Besides temporary causes, AF can be associated with permanent heart disease, such as valvular disease in which context AF is called valvular AF. Coronary heart disease, heart failure, hypertension, left ventricular hypertrophy, all forms of cardiomyopathies, and cardiac tumors have been associated with a high incidence of AF and carry a worse prognosis when compared to isolated form of AF. As mentioned, AF can occur in isolated or familial forms, without apparent identifiable underlying disease [3].

The main pathway for diagnosis of AF is through electrocardiographic record. A first-detected or recorded episode of AF is defined as the first one, despite the fact whether the patient was symptomatic or not and the possibility of the previous undetected episodes. Presentation of the patients with AF can differ, from with vague non-specific symptoms to thromboembolic consequences. Generally speaking, symptoms of AF depend of the rate of ventricular response, irregularity of the rhythm, functional status, duration of AF, and many more factors. As previously noted, the diagnosis of AF requires 12-lead electrocardiographic documentation or ambulatory Holter monitoring (especially in patients with daily paroxysms, but its usefulness is less in patients who have paroxysms at intervals more than 24 h). In patients with paroxysm with intervals that are greater than 24 h, implantable loop record devices, such as Reveal LINQ or CONFIRM, are used, as well as atrial high-rate episode recordings in patients with implantable dual-chamber pacemakers [1, 3].

2. Treatment strategies

Before initiating a treatment in patient with AF, we should first consider the probability of reoccurrence and/or persistence of the arrhythmia as well as patient symptomatology. Treatment strategies can be rate and rhythm control. For rhythm control, antiarrhythmic drugs, direct current cardioversion, and electrophysiological ablation are used, while for rate control, chronotropic drugs are being used, while AV node ablation is required in order to reduce rapid ventricular rate response which is often observed in patients with AF.

2.1 Rhythm control strategy

The rhythm control strategy implies the use of cardioversion to convert AF to normal, sinus rhythm. Cardioversion can be either pharmacological or electrical. Depending on the factors that lead to AF, not all attempts of cardioversion are successful, with about 50% of patients reverting to AF within a year of cardioversion [10]. Pharmacological cardioversion is preferred over electrical, especially in patients who present with AF within 48 h, while electrical is a standard procedure for AF with duration of more than 48 h. Rhythm control strategy by using antiarrhythmic drugs is an essential part in management of AF whose goals are prevention of reoccurrence and modification of recurrences by making them less symptomatic, less frequent, and less sustained [3].

Patients with persistent AF should be considered for either pharmacological or direct current cardioversion (DCCV) despite symptomatology, unless there are contraindications. Antiarrhythmic drugs may be prescribed to patients before and/or after successful DCCV for a period of time in order to prevent reoccurrence of AF. The use of antiarrhythmic drugs before DC conversion can also improve successfulness of DC conversion by prolongation of atrial refractoriness [11]. Besides antiarrhythmic drugs, patients may also require antithrombotic therapy. The recommendations for anticoagulation therapy are the same for both pharmacological and electrical cardioversion.

Antiarrhythmic drugs express their effect by blocking ion channels by which they affect atrial or junctional automaticity or refractoriness. By this mechanism, antiarrhythmic drugs suppress the trigger of AF (frequent atrial premature beats, rapid atrial tachycardia, etc.). Besides that, these drugs decrease excitability and conduction velocity by discouraging reentry mechanism or by changing autonomic stimulation (such as beta-blockers).

Side effect profiles, safety, and underlying heart diseases and their nature influence the choice of antiarrhythmic drugs; however, drugs with the greatest effects are also the ones that have bigger proarrhythmic effects and negative inotropic effects.

In the most cases, optimal beta-blockade represents the first line or is already administered for underlying heart diseases or for ventricular rate control in AF. If beta-blockers fail in rhythm control strategy or are contraindicated, a specific antiarrhythmic drug may be used. The selection of specific antiarrhythmic drug depends mostly on associated cardiovascular disease. Typically, patients can be divided into four categories: those with no or minimal heart disease, hypertensive heart (with or without significant left ventricular hypertrophy), ischemic heart disease, and heart failure. Also, besides this classification, patients can also be divided into two categories according to the presence of heart failure with reduced ejection fraction (ejection fraction <35%) or not (ejection fraction >35%) [1].

In patients with no or minimal heart disease, generally flecainide and propafenone are the first-line drugs. Dofetilide and dronedarone are the second-line drugs; since monitoring is required and expenses are high, amiodarone is reserved as the last-line therapy, while sotalol is being avoided because of the need for hospitalization and acquired long QT syndrome. **Figure 1** shows the optimal choice of antiarrhythmic drugs according to the underlying heart disease.

For patients who have left ventricular hypertrophy and AF, only two drugs are available: dronedarone and amiodarone. Thus, in patients with severe hypertrophy, there is only sufficient clinical experience with amiodarone. Sotalol and dofetilide should be avoided in the presence of significant left ventricular hypertrophy, since there is significant risk of QT prolongation and development of malignant arrhythmias. Antiarrhythmics of class Ic (propafenone and flecainide) are also not used because of proarrhythmic effect.

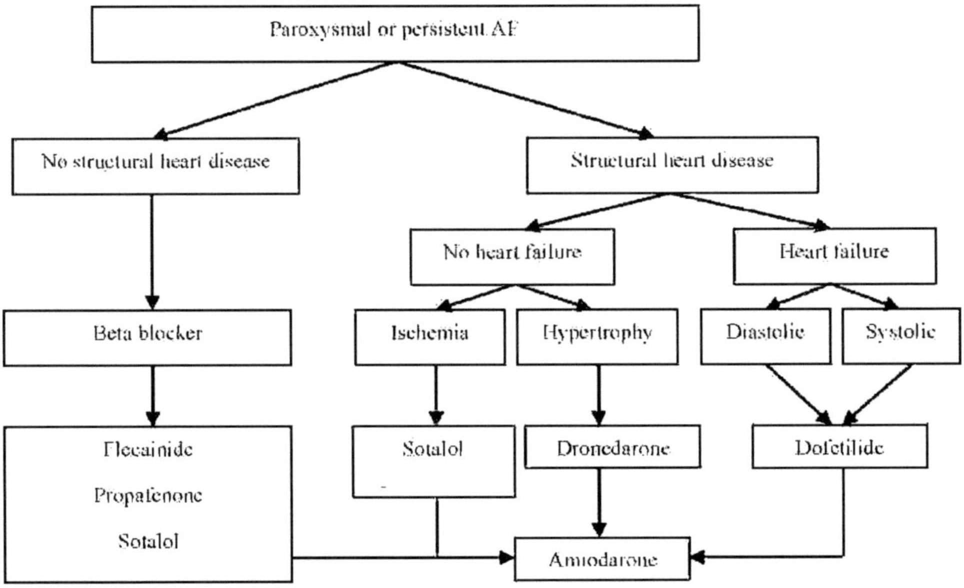

Figure 1.
Optimal choice of antiarrhythmic drug in different clinical settings [modified from Shenasa and Camm [1]].

Patients with coronary artery disease and paroxysmal or persistent AF should be treated with sotalol, amiodarone, or dronedarone, since they are both anti-ischemic and antiarrhythmic; however, sometimes sotalol and dronedarone are avoided because of proarrhythmic risk or progression to permanent AF. Propafenone and flecainide are contraindicated in patients with coronary artery disease since increased mortality was observed in the Cardiac Arrhythmia Suppression Trial (CAST) in patients with post-myocardial infarction with active ischemia [12].

For patients with heart failure and paroxysmal and persistent AF, only amiodarone and dronedarone can be considered for all grades of heart failure. However, dronedarone should be avoided in patients with recently unstable New York Heart Association (NYHA) class IV heart failure, particularly in patients with ejection fraction of left ventricle less than 35%. Even though there is no or little alternative to amiodarone for patients with heart failure in Europe, there are some concerns regarding the use of amiodarone in NYHA class III heart failure.

For acute pharmacological cardioversion, oral or intravenous antiarrhythmics with class Ic (flecainide and propafenone) or III (amiodarone, ibutilide, and dofetilide) can be used or new, atrial selective agent—vernakalant [3]. Depending on the agent as well as factors that lead to the development of AF, the rate of successful conversion to normal, sinus rhythm differs [13]. Out-of-hospital conversion of AF can also be achieved in patients with persistent AF with pill-in-the-pocket strategy which consists of self-administration of single oral dose of class Ic antiarrhythmics on the onset of symptoms of AF.

Assessment of rhythm control strategy should not be led by the presence or absence of symptoms since many clinical trials concluded that there is often little or no association between symptoms and reoccurrence of AF; therefore, prolonged monitoring is advised. In situation where patient is adequately anticoagulated, frequent visits are not necessary; however, if the initiation of anticoagulation therapy is based on the frequency of arrhythmia episodes, detailed and prolonged monitoring is required (24 h ECG Holter monitoring, 48 h ECG Holter monitoring, 7-day ECG Holter monitoring or implantable loop recorded implantation).

2.2 Rate control strategy

In patients with permanent AF, control of the ventricular response rate is important, since a lot research suggested that high heart rates were associated with poor outcomes in the terms of mortality. Besides patients with permanent AF, the rate control strategy should be also implied for the patients with paroxysmal AF when relapse occurs, especially if the patients are symptomatic or hemodynamically compromised by it. Rapid ventricular rates can cause palpitations or even a syncope and other rate-related symptoms; however, these high ventricular rates lead to degradation of left ventricle performance, mitral regurgitation, and further dilatation of the left atrium. If the heart rate exceeds 125 beats per minute, even a normal ventricle may dilate, but in patients with impaired left ventricle function, even less heart rates can cause further dilatation. On the other hand, the loss of atrial contraction (observed in patients with AF), which approximately accounts for 20–30% of the total stroke volume of left ventricle, leads to further reduction in cardiac output. Besides these two mechanisms, irregularity in ventricle rhythm additionally impairs left ventricle function. That is why the goal of rate control strategy is heart rate below 115 beats per minute in light and/or moderate physical activity and below 80 beats per minute in rest. However, sometimes ventricle rates at rest do not adequately represent effective control during exercise [1, 14].

Principles of rate control strategy may be easy to implement in patients with permanent AF and then in those with paroxysmal or persistent form since the control of the heart rate in arrhythmia and in sinus rhythm can and are often different, especially in patients with dysfunction of sinus node. In these circumstances, symptomatic bradycardia with long sinus pauses can occur. In these patients, heart rate support is needed, and implantation of dual-chamber pacemaker is often needed. Therefore, the main reason for rate control strategy in patients with intermittent AF is failure to find adequate blend of the effect on heart rate during AF and when sinus rhythm occurs. It should be noted that effects of different antiarrhythmic drugs have different effects on AV node, whereas beta-blockers have less marked effect on AV node than calcium channel blockers and cause sinus bradycardia more often.

Three different classes of drugs are being used for rate control: digitalis, calcium channel blockers, and beta-blockers. Beta-blockers and calcium channel blockers are preferred over digitalis and should be used in most of the patients with chronic AF without heart failure, while in patients with chronic AF and heart failure, digoxin or amiodarone should be used in order to control ventricular rate. By using digitalis, adequate control of exercise heart rate is rarely achieved, so in patients who are mildly to moderately physically active, there will be no benefit. Digitalis is also less efficacious than amiodarone and calcium channel blockers and in some studies even beta-blockers. Most patients should be treated with beta-blocker (usually beta-2 specific beta-blocker like bisoprolol, metoprolol, carvedilol, or nebivolol) or calcium channel blocker with rate-limiting effect, such as verapamil or diltiazem. In patients whom adequate control of heart rate is not achieved, a combination of drugs is needed; however, it is not advised in patients with reduced left ventricle function. Amiodarone is reserved as a last-line therapy, especially for patients with heart failure and with reduced ejection fraction. It is a powerful and very effective heart rate-limiting drug, but many adverse effects are the main drawback of amiodarone therapy [15–18] .

Besides traditional therapy for rate control, in patients with AF and in whom rate is not adequately achieved, the use of sotalol and amiodarone can slow the AV conduction, but they are not commonly used for long-term rate control because of the proarrhythmic risk. In situations where rapid control of heart rate is needed, oral administration is not feasible, but intravenous administration of diltiazem can be considered, while in patients without heart failure or accessory pathways, intravenous beta-blockers (esmolol, metoprolol, and propranolol), diltiazem, and verapamil may be used. If the patient has accessory pathway, only intravenous amiodarone is indicated [3].

The doses of drugs used for rate control strategy are given in **Table 1** [1].

If the rate control cannot be established, interventional approach can also be performed by ablation of AV node/His bundle alongside with implantation of pacemaker.

For the assessment of rate control strategy, palpation of the radial pulse with auscultation of heart murmurs, and electrocardiography can be easily obtained and provide sufficient information for most of the patients. If needed, 6 min walk test or 24 h ambulatory Holter ECG monitoring can be implemented giving more reliable information regarding resting and exercise heart rate.

2.3 Direct current cardioversion

Prior to DC conversion it is important to evaluate each patient for appropriateness, maintaining normal, sinus rhythm thereafter, as well as probability of successful cardioversion [3]. Several factors can influence success of the cardioversion and/or reoccurrence of AF, such as age, underlying valve disease, duration of AF, size of the left atrium, low functional class, and possibility of concomitant administration of antiarrhythmic drugs. DC cardioversion has been extensively used with vitamin K-dependent anticoagulants (VKAs), while more recently direct oral anticoagulants (DOACs) have been also used for thromboembolic prevention in patients who are undergoing DC conversion.

DC cardioversion is being performed short-acting general anesthetics or under heavy sedation, while assessment of potassium levels and therapeutic levels of digoxin is indicated in all patients, since hypokalemia and supratherapeutic levels of digoxin can precipitate ventricular arrhythmias in patients with DC cardioversion. Synchronization is used to avoid discharging on T waves since it can result in ventricular arrhythmias.

Drug	Average dose	Clinical setting	Adverse effects
Digoxin	Loading dose: 250 mcg every 2 h; up to 1500 mcg Maintenance dose: 125–250 mcg daily	As monotherapy in elderly patients; not physically active patients	Bradycardia; AV blocks; proarrhythmic
Bisoprolol	5–10 mg daily	Patients with coronary artery disease; heart failure	Hypotension; bradycardia, especially in paroxysmal AF; AV blocks; impairment of pulmonary function in chronic obstructive pulmonary disease or asthma
Metoprolol	50–200 mg daily		
Carvedilol	25–100 mg daily		
Nebivolol	5–10 mg daily		
Sotalol	80–320 mg daily	Recurrent AF	Not recommended in permanent AF; bradycardia; QT prolongation; proarrhythmic
Verapamil	80–360 mg daily	Patients with chronic obstructive pulmonary disease and asthma	Hypotension; AV blocks; heart failure
Diltiazem	120–360 mg daily		
Amiodarone	200 mg daily	Recurrent AF; heart failure	Bradycardia; AV blocks; QT prolongation; proarrhythmic

Table 1.
Average doses of antiarrhythmic drugs used for rate control in AF [1].

If monophasic DC cardioversion is being used, an initial 300 J biphasic shock or 150 J monophasic shock should be given, followed by the second 200 J monophasic or 300 J biphasic shock if the first one fails. If the second shock fails, the third and final one can be delivered with the same magnitude as the second one. Biphasic shocks at high output are more successful than monophasic shocks at the same output [3].

2.4 Ablation strategies

Currently, the main way of nonpharmacological rhythm control is catheter ablation of AF, without the risk of long-term antiarrhythmic therapy maintaining normal, sinus rhythm. It has been shown that catheter ablation significantly improves LV function, symptoms, exercise capacity, and quality of life. In addition, some meta-analyses have shown that catheter ablation was superior to antiarrhythmic drugs for the control of AF. The benefit of catheter ablation was even greater in paroxysmal AF when compared to medical therapy [18]. Catheter ablation was also better than antiarrhythmics in terms of higher rates of freedom from both AF and antiarrhythmic medications [19]. However, no mortality benefit was observed in patients who have undergone catheter ablation of AF, so the procedure is currently reserved for patients with symptomatic AF [20].

Besides catheter ablation, one more way of treatment of AF includes surgical ablation of AF. The procedure involves creating series of incisions in both the left and the right atria, by which propagation of sinus impulse is directed through both atria and at the same time disabling multiple macro-reentrant circuits. Currently, the standard surgical technique has been replaced with linear epicardial ablation using unipolar or bipolar radiofrequency ablation, cryoablation, laser, high-frequency ultrasound, and microwave energy. Also, surgical instrumentation now enables minimally invasive approaches through mini-thoracotomies with video assistance. Stand-alone surgical and epicardial AF ablation may be considered for patients who are symptomatic and were refractory to one or more attempts of catheter ablation or for patients who are not candidates for catheter ablation. Hence, there are no studies that compared effects of surgical and catheter ablation of AF, degree of patient discomfort, longer hospitalizations, and the risk of bleeding following left atrial appendage excision, patients prefer catheter ablation to surgical [20].

2.5 Anticoagulant therapy

Anticoagulation therapy is one of the cornerstones in management of patients with AF, since the most common consequence of AF is stroke.

The recommendations for anticoagulation therapy are the same for both pharmacological and electrical cardioversion. CHA_2DS_2-VASc risk score is being used in order to assess whether the patient is in need for anticoagulation therapy, while HAS-BLED score assesses the risk of bleeding in patients on anticoagulation therapy. Anticoagulation therapy can be either with the use of direct oral anticoagulants (DOACs), such as apixaban, rivaroxaban, dabigatran, or edoxaban, or the use of vitamin K-dependent anticoagulants (VKAs) such as warfarin and acenocumarol. In patient with VKAs, assessment of INR is very important and should always be within 2.0–3.0 unless there are other cofactors (mechanical valves, etc.).

3. Pharmacology of antiarrhythmic drugs

The choice of antiarrhythmic drug and its superiority of one over another are not well investigated due to many reasons, such as enrolment of patients with different underlying heart diseases or suboptimal design. Doses, indications, and the main adverse effects of the most commonly used antiarrhythmics are given in **Table 2** [1].

3.1 Flecainide and propafenone

As antiarrhythmic drugs of class Ic, propafenone and flecainide are frequently used for rhythm control in patients with AF and no or minimal underlying heart disease (such as heart failure, left ventricular hypertrophy, coronary artery disease, or previous myocardial infarction).

Flecainide expresses its effect with potent blockade of sodium and potassium channels, however, not prolonging the QT interval.

Propafenone has similar effects as quinidine, although it possesses some beta-blocking activity without prolonging the action potential.

In clinical trials that investigated recurrence rates, both propafenone and flecainide reduced the recurrence rate by 70%. Co-administration of AV-slowing agents such as beta-blockers is advised because of the possibility of organization of AF into atrial flutter. When directly compared, there was no superiority of propafenone over flecainide [21].

Drug	Dose	Clinical setting	Adverse effects
Flecainide	100–200 mg two times per day	Minimal or no structural heart disease	Bradycardia; AV blocks; organization into atrial flutter; deterioration of renal function
Flecainide XL	200 mg one time per day		
Propafenone	150–300 mg three times per day		Bradycardia; AV blocks; organization into atrial flutter; new onset of myocardial ischemia; metallic taste
Propafenone SR	225–425 mg two times per day		
Sotalol	80–160 mg two times per day	Stable coronary artery disease without previous myocardial infarction; hypertension without significant left ventricle hypertrophy	Bradycardia; AV blocks; proarrhythmic; potassium level disorders
Dofetilide	125–500 mcg two times per day	Previous myocardial infarction; heart failure	Torsade de pontes; bradycardia; AV blocks; proarrhythmic
Amiodarone	100–200 mg one time per day	Heart failure; hypertrophic cardiomyopathy; significant left ventricular hypertrophy	Bradycardia; AV blocks; thyrotoxic; pulmonary fibrosis; hepatic toxicity; eye toxicity, skin rash; abdominal pain; peripheral edema; dyspnea
Dronedarone	400 mg two times per day	Heart failure NYHA I–II; coronary artery disease; left ventricular hypertrophy	Bradycardia; AV blocks; diarrhea; rash

Table 2.
Doses, indications, and adverse effects of the most commonly used antiarrhythmic drugs [1].

3.2 Beta-blockers

The most effective antiarrhythmic drugs in prevention of AF are considered as beta-blockers. Even though they are mainly used in rate control strategy, in AF caused by thyrotoxicosis, after cardiac surgery or any adrenergically mediated AF, they represent the first-choice therapy. Between the groups of beta-blockers, there is limited evidence of superiority of one over another. Some, such as carvedilol, may be more potent because of synergistic effect on ion channels as well as adrenergic blockade; however, in direct comparison to bisoprolol, no benefit was observed [22, 23].

3.3 Sotalol

Sotalol, an antiarrhythmic drug of class III and beta-blocker, offers additional benefit of slowing heart rate during reoccurrences in AF episodes. It is recommended for use in patients with AF and stable coronary artery disease without previous myocardial infarction and/or dysfunction of the left ventricle and patients with AF and hypertension without significant left ventricle hypertrophy.

When compared with amiodarone, it showed inferior results with 30% of patients remaining in sinus rhythm after 2 years of therapy, while in the group of amiodarone, 60% remained in sinus rhythm. In comparison with antiarrhythmics class Ic, it showed similar effects [24–26].

Bradycardia and hypotension represent the most common side effects, while prolongation of QT with proarrhythmic effect was less common. Due to its relatively simple pharmacokinetics, it has very few drug interactions; however, it should be noted that sotalol decreases the threshold for cardiac defibrillation.

3.4 Dofetilide

Dofetilide is also one of the antiarrhythmic drugs of class III, but unlike sotalol or antiarrhythmics class Ic, it is recommended for use in patients with previous myocardial infarction and in patients with heart failure. It does not produce blockade of other potassium or sodium channels, but the rate of recovery from the blockade is slow; therefore, the extent of blockade shows little dependence on stimulation frequency.

Dofetilide has a dose-dependent effect; increased dose resulted in increased proportion of patients converted to sinus rhythm. However it comes with the cost. Its major concern is development of torsade de pontes which is also dose-related and often occurs in the first days after dofetilide initiation; therefore, in-hospital initiation is mandatory. Treatment with dofetilide should be initiated based on the rate-corrected QT interval (QTc) and serum electrolytes. A baseline QTc greater than 450 ms, bradycardia with heart rate less than 50 beats per minute, and hypokalemia are relative contraindications.

Since 80% of oral dose is being eliminated unchanged by the kidneys and its dose-related side effects, dofetilide dosage must be based on the estimated creatinine clearance [27].

3.5 Amiodarone

Amiodarone is one of the most commonly used antiarrhythmic worldwide, as a result of its broad spectrum of antiarrhythmic action.

Amiodarone markedly prolongs the duration of action potential, thus prolonging the QT interval. Despite its belonging to class III of antiarrhythmics, it also blocks inactivated sodium channels and has weak adrenergic and calcium channel blocking effect by which it slows down heart rate and AV node conduction.

It has great potential to maintain sinus rhythm in patients with underlying cardiovascular conditions. Its effect on rhythm control has been largely investigated; however, one main drawback of amiodarone use is its side effects. Looking on proarrhythmic effects, it has low potential to induce torsade de pontes; however, non-cardiac side effects are numerous. It did not show effect on all-cause mortality; however, it can be used in management of AF in clinical settings of heart failure, hypertrophic cardiomyopathy, and significant left ventricular hypertrophy caused by hypertension [28].

Amiodarone side effects are a result of dose and accumulation in many tissues (lungs, liver, skin, and even heart). It also blocks the peripheral conversion of thyroxine to triiodothyronine and may result in hyperthyroidism and hypothyroidism, which in many cases are the most frequent side effects.

3.6 Dronedarone

Besides sotalol, dofetilide, and amiodarone, dronedarone is also a member of class III of antiarrhythmic and has been widely used in prevention of recurrence of paroxysmal or persistent AF and is also effective in slowing ventricular rated during AF.

It is structural analog of amiodarone in which iodine atoms have been removed, therefore eliminating action on thyroxine metabolism.

Large clinical trials have demonstrated that dronedarone reduced relative risk of hospitalizations due to cardiovascular causes and death, differed the time to the first hospitalization for cardiovascular disease or death from any cause, and significantly reduced deaths from cardiovascular diseases [29]. Based on the antiarrhythmic trial with dronedarone in moderate to severe heart failure evaluating morbidity decrease (ANDROMEDA) study with patients with severe congestive heart failure, which was stopped ahead of time because excess death was revealed in dronedarone group, dronedarone should not be used in patients with severe heart failure [30]. Therefore, dronedarone is currently recommended for use in patients with paroxysmal AF with reducing the need of hospitalization for cardiovascular events or after conversion of persistent AF; however, it should be avoided in patients with permanent AF or advanced heart failure (**Table 3**).

3.7 Other antiarrhythmics

Ranolazine, an antianginal agent, belongs to more recently developed antiarrhythmics or recently investigated as antiarrhythmic drug. It blocks several ion channels and foremost on atrial level. Clinical investigations have demonstrated that it has potential to facilitate electrical cardioversion in refractory patients, efficacy as the pill-in-the-pocket approach, and enhancing pharmacological cardioversion with its synergistic effect with amiodarone [31, 32]. When combined with dronedarone, it also showed promising results [33]. However, further studies are needed to explore its full antiarrhythmic potential.

Vernakalant is relatively a new antiarrhythmic drug, and its main effect is achieved by blocking the sodium channels. Besides sodium channels it also blocks other channels and mild QT interval prolongation. Besides oral, vernakalant can also be administered intravenously, making it a preferable choice for rapid conversion of AF. It has been investigated for converting recent-onset AF. In some clinical trials, it showed superior efficacy when compared to amiodarone for acute conversion of AF [34]. It is recommended in patients with AF and no or minimal ischemic or structural heart disease and may be considered in patients with AF and mild to

Vaughan-Williams class		Mechanism of action	Drug	Dose	Clinical setting	Adverse effects
I class	*Ia class*	Moderate blockade of sodium channels	*Quinidine*	200–600 mg three times per day	Brugada syndrome; atrial fibrillation and flutter as last-line drug	Diarrhea; prolongation of QTc; enhances digitalis toxicity; proarrhythmic
			Disopyramide	400–800 mg two to three times per day	Ventricular arrhythmias	Proarrhythmic; dry mouth; blurred vision; hypotension; increased incidence of heart failure
	Ib class	Weak blockade of sodium channels	*Lidocaine*	1–1.5 mg/kg i.v.	Ventricular arrhythmias in acute myocardial infarction	Hypotension; edema; methemoglobinemia
			Mexiletine	200–300 mg three times per day	Ventricular arrhythmias	Proarrhythmic; bradycardia; AV blocks
	Ic class	Strong blockade of sodium channels	*Flecainide*	100–200 mg two times per day	Minimal or no structural heart disease	Bradycardia; AV blocks; organization into atrial flutter; deterioration of renal function
			Propafenone	150–300 mg three times per day		Bradycardia; AV blocks; organization into atrial flutter; new onset of myocardial ischemia; metallic taste
II class		Beta 1 selective	*Bisoprolol*	5–10 mg daily	Patients with coronary artery disease; heart failure	Hypotension; bradycardia, especially in paroxysmal AF; AV blocks; impairment of pulmonary function in chronic obstructive pulmonary disease or asthma
		Beta 1 selective	*Metoprolol*	50–200 mg daily		
		Nonselective	*Carvedilol*	25–100 mg daily		
		Strong beta 1 selectivity and vasodilatation	*Nebivolol*	5–10 mg daily		
III class		Blockade of potassium channels and increasing effective refractory period	*Sotalol*	80–320 mg daily	Stable coronary artery disease without previous myocardial infarction; hypertension without significant left ventricle hypertrophy	Bradycardia; AV blocks; proarrhythmic; potassium level disorders

Vaughan-Williams class	Mechanism of action	Drug	Dose	Clinical setting	Adverse effects
		Dofetilide	125–500 mcg two times per day	Previous myocardial infarction; heart failure	Torsade de pontes; bradycardia; AV blocks; proarrhythmic;
		Amiodarone	100–200 mg one time per day	Heart failure; hypertrophic cardiomyopathy; significant left ventricular hypertrophy	Bradycardia; AV blocks; thyrotoxic; pulmonary fibrosis; hepatic toxicity; eye toxicity, skin rash, abdominal pain; peripheral edema; dyspnea
		Dronedarone	400 mg two times per day	Heart failure NYHA I–II; coronary artery disease; left ventricular hypertrophy	Bradycardia; AV blocks; diarrhea; rash
IV class	Slow non-dihydropyridine calcium channel blockers	*Verapamil*	80–360 mg daily	Patients with chronic obstructive pulmonary disease and asthma	Hypotension; AV blocks; heart failure
		Diltiazem	120–360 mg daily		

Table 3.
Antiarrhythmic drugs, Vaughan-Williams class, mechanism of action, doses, clinical settings, and adverse effects [1].

moderate structural heart disease as well as post-cardiac surgery AF. It is also more effective than flecainide and propafenone, again in recent-onset AF, and is well tolerated while to most common side effects including paresthesia, dysgeusia, dizziness, sneezing, and nausea [35, 36].

4. Conclusions

AF represents as one of the most common cardiovascular diseases and a major cause of stroke in developed countries. Treatment strategies can be divided into two strategies: rate and rhythm control. For rhythm control, antiarrhythmic drugs, direct current cardioversion, and electrophysiological ablation are used, while for rate control, chronotropic drugs are being used, while AV node ablation is required in order to reduce rapid ventricular rate which is often observed in patients with AF. **Table 3** summarizes all antiarrhythmics with Vaughan-Williams class, mechanism of action, doses, clinical settings, and adverse effects.

Patients with paroxysmal or persistent form of AF should be considered for either pharmacological or DC despite symptomatology, unless there are contraindications. Rapid ventricular rates can cause palpitations or even a syncope and other rate-related symptoms; however, these high ventricular rates lead to degradation of left ventricle performance, mitral regurgitation, and further dilatation of the left atrium; therefore, if the conversion is not achievable, patients should be treated with rate control strategy.

Conflict of interest

The authors declare no conflict of interest.

Acronyms and abbreviations

AF	atrial fibrillation
DC	direct current cardioversion
NYHA	New York Heart Association classification
DOAC	direct oral anticoagulants
VKA	vitamin K-dependent anticoagulants
QTc	corrected QT interval

Author details

Stefan Simović[1,2*], Ivan Srejović[3], Vladimir Živković[3], Slobodanka Mitrović[4,5], Jovana Jeremić[6], Vladimir Jakovljević[3,7] and Goran Davidović[1,2]

1 Department of Internal Medicine, Faculty of Medical Sciences, University of Kragujevac, Kragujevac, Serbia

2 Clinic for Cardiology, Clinical Center Kragujevac, Kragujevac, Serbia

3 Department of Physiology, Faculty of Medical Sciences, University of Kragujevac, Kragujevac, Serbia

4 Department of Pathology, Faculty of Medical Sciences, University of Kragujevac, Kragujevac, Serbia

5 Department of Pathology, Clinical Center Kragujevac, Kragujevac, Serbia

6 Department of Pharmacology, Faculty of Medical Sciences, University of Kragujevac, Kragujevac, Serbia

7 Department of Human Pathology, 1st Moscow State Medical University IM Sechenov, Moscow, Russia

*Address all correspondence to: simovicst@gmail.com

References

[1] Shenasa M, Camm JA. Management of Atrial Fibrillation: A Practical Approach. 1st ed. Oxford: Oxford University Press; 2015. pp. 1-83. ISBN: 978-0-19-968631-5

[2] Barrios V, Calderón A, Escobar C, de la Figuera M. Patients with atrial fibrilladion in a primary care setting: Val-FAAP study [en representación del Grupo de Atención Primaria de la sección de Cardiología Clínica de la Sociedad Española de Cardiología]. Revista Española de Cardiología. 2012;**65**(1):47-53

[3] Yap YG, Camm JA. Essentials of Atrial Fibrillation. 2nd ed. London: Springer Healthcare; 2014. pp. 1-34. DOI: 10.1007/978-1-907673-98-6_3

[4] Allesie M, Lammers WJEP, Bonke FIM, Hollen J. Experimental evaluation of Moe's multiple wavelet hypothesis of atrial fibrillation. In: Zipes DP, Jalife J, editors. Cardiac Electrophysiology and Arrhythmias. Orlando, FL: Grune & Stratton INC; 1985. pp. 265-275

[5] Moe GKRW, Abildskov JA. A computer model of atrial fibrillation. American Heart Journal. 1964;**67**:200-220

[6] Haissaguerre M, Jais P, Shah DC, et al. Spontaneous initiation of atrial fibrillation by ectopic beats originating in the pulmonary veins. The New England Journal of Medicine. 1998;**339**:659-666

[7] Mandapati R, Skanes A, Chen J, et al. Stable microreentrant sources as a mechanism of atrial fibrillation in the isolated sheep heart. Circulation. 2000;**101**:194-199

[8] Skanes AC, Mandapati R, Berenfeld O, et al. Spatiotemporal periodicity during atrial fibrillation in the isolated sheep heart. Circulation. 1998;**98**:1236-1248

[9] Fioranelli M, Piccoli M, Mileto GM, et al. Analysis of heart rate variability five minutes before the onset of paroxysmal atrial fibrillation. Pacing and Clinical Electrophysiology. 1999;**22**:743-749

[10] Lim H, Hamaad A, Lip G. Clinical review: Clinical management of atrial fibrillation—Rate control versus rhythm control. Critical Care. 2004;**8**:271-279

[11] Meurling CJ, Roijer A, Waktare JE, Holmgvist F, Lindholm CJ, Ingemansson MP, et al. Prediction of sinus rhythm maintenance following DC-cardioversion of persistent atrial fibrillation—The role of atrial cycle length. BMC Cardiovascular Disorders. 2006;**6**:11

[12] Echt DS, Liebson PR, Mitchell LB, Peters RW, Obias-Manno D, Barker AH, et al. Mortality and morbidity in patients receiving encainide, flecainide, or placebo. The cardiac arrhythmia suppression trial. The New England Journal of Medicine. 1991;**324**:781-788

[13] Camm AJ. Safety considerations in the pharmacological management of atrial fibrillation. International Journal of Cardiology. 2008;**127**:299-306

[14] Van Gelder IC, Wyse DG, Chandler ML, Cooper HA, Olshansky B, Hagens VE, et al. Does intensity of rate-control influence outcome in atrial fibrillation? An analysis of pooled data from the RACE and AFFIRM studies. Europace. 2006;**8**:935-942

[15] Farshi R, Kistner D, Sarma JS, Longmate JA, Singh BN. Ventricular rate control in chronic atrial fibrillation during daily activity and programmed exercise: A crossover open-label study of five drug regimens. Journal of the

American College of Cardiology. 1999;**33**:304-310

[16] Khand AU, Rankin AC, Martin W, Taylor J, Gemmell I, Cleland JG. Carvedilol alone or in combination with digoxin for the management of atrial fibrillation in patients with heart failure? Journal of the American College of Cardiology. 2003;**42**:1944-1951

[17] Olshansky B, Rosenfeld LE, Warner AL, Solomon AJ, O'Neill G, Sharma A, et al. The atrial fibrillation follow-up investigation of rhythm management (AFFIRM) study: Approaches to control rate in atrial fibrillation. Journal of the American College of Cardiology. 2004;**43**:1201-1208

[18] Rosso R, Sparks PB, Morton JB, et al. Vagal paroxysmal atrial fibrillation: Prevalence and ablation outcome in patients without structural heart disease. Journal of Cardiovascular Electrophysiology. 2010;**21**:489-493

[19] Khan MN, Jais P, Cummings J, et al. Pulmonary-vein isolation for atrial fibrillation in patients with heart failure. The New England Journal of Medicine. 2008;**359**:1778-1785

[20] Issa ZF, Miller JM, Zipes DP. Clinical Arrhythmology and Electrophysiology. 2nd ed. Philadelphia, PA: Elsevier Saunders; 2012. pp. 307-310. ISBN: 978-1-4557-1274-8

[21] Chimienti M, Cullen MT Jr, Casadei G. Safety of long-term flecainide and propafenone in the management of patients with symptomatic paroxysmal atrial fibrillation: Report from the flecainide and propafenone Italian study investigators. The American Journal of Cardiology. 1996;**77**:60A-75A

[22] Kühlkamp V, Schirdewan A, Stangl K, Homberg M, Ploch M, Beck OA. Use of metoprolol CR/XL to maintain sinus rhythm after conversion from persistent atrial fibrillation: A randomized, double-blind, placebo-controlled study. Journal of the American College of Cardiology. 2000;**36**:139-146

[23] Katritsis DG, Panagiotakos DB, Karvouni E, Giazitzoglou E, Korovesis S, Paxinos G, et al. Comparison of effectiveness of carvedilol versus bisoprolol for maintenance of sinus rhythm after cardioversion of persistent atrial fibrillation. The American Journal of Cardiology. 2003;**92**:1116-1119

[24] Roy D, Talajic M, Dorian P, Connolly S, Eisenberg MJ, Green M, et al. Amiodarone to prevent recurrence of atrial fibrillation. The New England Journal of Medicine. 2000;**342**:913-920

[25] Singh BN, Singh SN, Reda DJ, Tang XC, Lopez B, Harris CL, et al. Amiodarone versus sotalol for atrial fibrillation. The New England Journal of Medicine. 2005;**352**:1861-1872

[26] The AFFIRM First Antiarrhythmic Drug Substudy Investigators. Maintenance of sinus rhythm in patients with atrial fibrillation: An AFFIRM substudy of first antiarrhythmic drug. Journal of the American College of Cardiology. 2003;**42**:20-29

[27] Katzung BG. Basic & Clinical Pharmacology. 14th ed. USA: McGraw-Hill Education. pp. 228-247. ISBN: 978-1-259-64115-2

[28] Bardy GH, Lee KL, Mark DB, Poole JE, Packer DL, Boineau R, et al. Amiodarone or an implantable cardioverter-defibrillator for congestive heart failure. The New England Journal of Medicine. 2005;**352**:225-237

[29] Singh BN, Connolly SJ, Crijns HJ, Roy D, Kowey PR, Capucci A, et al. Dronedarone for maintenance of sinus rhythm in atrial fibrillation or flutter.

The New England Journal of Medicine. 2007;**357**(10):978-999

[30] Køber L, Torp-Pedersen C, McMurray JJ, Gøtzsche O, Lévy S, Crijns H, et al. Increased mortality after dronedarone therapy for severe heart failure. The New England Journal of Medicine. 2008;**358**:2678-2687

[31] Murdock DK, Kersten M, Kaliebe J, Larrain G. The use of oral ranolazine to convert new or paroxysmal atrial fibrillation: A review of experience with implications for possible "pill in the pocket" approach to atrial fibrillation. Indian Pacing and Electrophysiology Journal. 2008;**9**:260-267

[32] Murdock DK, Reiffel JA, Kaliebe JW, Larrain G. The use of ranolazine to facilitate electrical cardioversion in cardioversion-resistant patients: A case series. Pacing and Clinical Electrophysiology. 2012;**35**:302-307

[33] Reiffel JA, Camm AJ, Belardinelli L, Zeng D, Karwatowska-Prokopczuk E, Olmsted A, et al. The HARMONY trial: Combined ranolazine and dronedarone in the management of paroxysmal atrial fibrillation: mechanistic and therapeutic synergism. Circulation. Arrhythmia and Electrophysiology. 2015;**8**(5):1048-1056

[34] Camm AJ, Capucci A, Hohnloser S, Torp-Pedersen C, Van Gelder IC, Mangal B, et al. A randomized active-controlled study comparing the efficacy and safety of vernakalant to amiodarone in recent onset atrial fibrillation. Journal of the American College of Cardiology. 2011;**57**:313-321

[35] Conde D, Costabel JP, Aragon M, Caro M, Ferro A, Klein A, et al. Flecainide or propafenone vs. vernakalant for conversion of recent-onset of atrial fibrillation. The Canadian Journal of Cardiology. 2013;**29**(10): 1330.e13

[36] Kossaify A. Vernakalant in atrial fibrillation: A relatively new weapon in the armamentarium against an old enemy. Drug Target Insights. 2019;**13**:1-7

Chapter 5

New Results in Catheter Ablation for Atrial Fibrillation

Nándor Szegedi and László Gellér

Abstract

Pulmonary vein isolation (PVI) is the cornerstone of rhythm-control therapy for atrial fibrillation (AF). A few years ago, contact force-sensing ablation catheters (CFSAC) were introduced. Nowadays the use of CFSAC became a part of the everyday practice. The durability of PVI depends much on the accurate lesion creation. The recently developed techniques (ablation index, CLOSE protocol) may facilitate the procedure in terms of achieving durable PVI which has already been confirmed by randomized trials. In this chapter, we would like to introduce the theoretical background of PVI and compare different techniques (radiofrequency point-by-point, cryoballoon, additional ablation lines for persistent AF) with special highlight on the importance of durable PVI.

Keywords: pulmonary vein isolation, atrial fibrillation, ablation, point-by-point, CLOSE protocol, cryoballoon

1. Introduction

Atrial fibrillation (AF) is the most common sustained arrhythmia. AF is associated with a higher risk of mortality than the general population [1]. It is one of the major causes of stroke, heart failure, sudden death, and cardiovascular morbidity in the world [2]. Thus, appropriate management of this arrhythmia and underlying diseases is of high importance. Besides stroke prevention with therapeutic anticoagulation, the rate-control or rhythm-control treatment is the basis of AF management.

Pulmonary vein isolation (PVI) is the cornerstone of rhythm-control therapy for atrial fibrillation [2, 3]. A few years ago, contact force-sensing ablation catheters (CFSAC) were introduced. Nowadays the use of CFSAC became a part of the everyday practice [4–8]. The durability of PVI depends much on the accurate lesion creation. The recently developed techniques (ablation index, CLOSE protocol) may facilitate the procedure in terms of achieving durable PVI which has already been confirmed by prospective trials [9–12]. In this chapter, we will introduce the theoretical background of PVI and compare different ablation techniques (radiofrequency point-by-point, cryoballoon, additional ablation lines for persistent AF) with special highlight on the importance of durable PVI.

2. Pulmonary vein isolation

2.1 Theoretical background of pulmonary vein isolation

The exact mechanism of atrial fibrillation for the individual patients is not well understood, and it is still a topic of intensive research nowadays. It seems that in most of the patients, the pulmonary veins and surrounding structures play an important role in the pathophysiology. The first cornerstone research was presented by Haissaguerre et al., where they found that electrical firing from the pulmonary veins (PVs) may have an important role in the initiation of atrial fibrillation paroxysms [13] (**Figure 1**).

Jais et al. showed distinctive electrophysiological properties of pulmonary veins in patients with AF compared with healthy patients' PVs. The main difference is the short or extremely short refractory period of the PVs which is likely to play a major role in the arrhythmogenesis [14]. Moreover, episodes of AF may shorten the effective refractory period of the atria and the PVs, which may promote recurrent and longer episodes of AF ("AF begets AF") [15, 16]. These studies are supplemented by another important finding by De Ponti et al. as they showed with high-density mapping of the PVs that majority of ectopic beats have a multifocal pattern and relatively proximal origin [17].

Besides the pulmonary veins, multiple pathophysiological factors may play a role in the mechanism of atrial fibrillation, like ligament of Marshall, vagal ganglia, micro-reentrant circuits, and spiral/rotational activities [18–21].

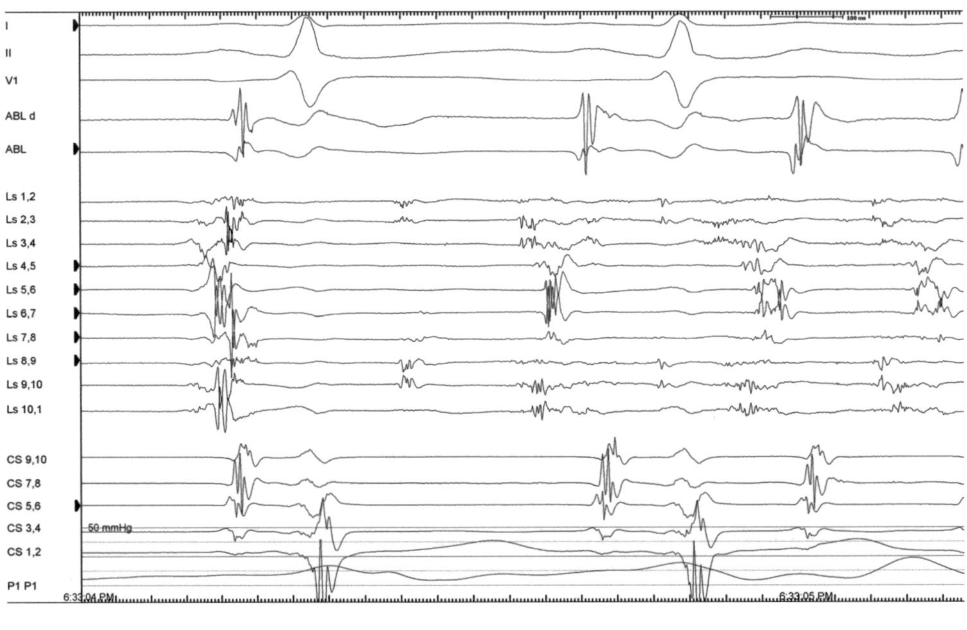

Figure 1.
High-frequency electrical activity in the right superior pulmonary vein registered on the Lasso (Ls) catheter.

2.2 Pulmonary vein isolation procedures

The two most frequently used ablation technologies for pulmonary vein isolation are radiofrequency point-by-point method which leads to coagulation necrosis by heating and single-shot cryoballoon ablation which leads to tissue necrosis by freezing.

PVI with radiofrequency ablation requires limited use of fluoroscopy, because catheter guidance is achieved with the use of an electroanatomical mapping system, but the approach requires extensive training due to the need for a more sophisticated catheter manipulation.

PVI with cryoballoon requires more extensive fluoroscopic guidance to position the balloon catheter at the pulmonary veins. On the other hand, the cryoballoon was developed to create a circular lesion around each pulmonary vein in a relatively simple manner, and thus it is less operator dependent.

Circumferential ablation around the PVs may have ablation-related benefits beyond pulmonary vein isolation, including concomitant ganglionated plexus modification and modification of other substrates located near the PVs [22].

2.2.1 Cryoballoon ablation

Pulmonary vein isolation can be reached with a balloon catheter by the occlusion of the pulmonary veins, causing tissue necrosis via cryothermal energy around antral orifice of the vessels. Occlusion of the pulmonary vein by the cryoballoon is tested by means of contrast injection and fluoroscopic examination (**Figure 2**). If the injection of contrast agent verifies the accurate occlusion of the pulmonary vein ostium, the freezing can be started. The need for fluoroscopic imaging for each PVs may contribute to a prolonged fluoroscopic time and dose.

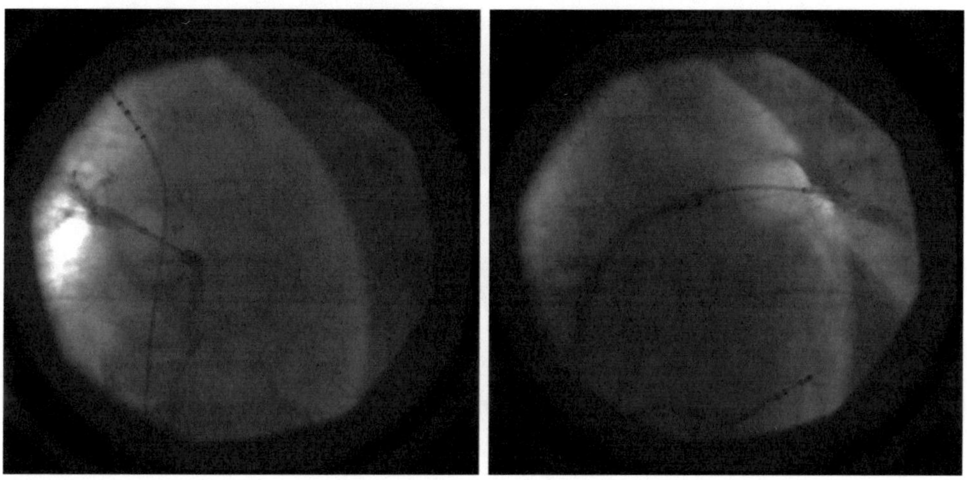

Figure2.
Right side: contrast injection in the right inferior pulmonary vein; decapolar catheter is placed in the superior vena cava to perform phrenic nerve pacing. Left side: contrast injection in the left superior pulmonary vein; decapolar catheter is placed in the coronary sinus.

First-generation cryoballoons deliver ablation only via the equator of the balloon. Freeze AF randomized trial found that first-generation cryoballoon was non-inferior as compared with the radiofrequency ablation. There was a higher rate of adverse events driven by the higher incidence of transient phrenic nerve palsy [23].

Second-generation cryoballoons were introduced to overcome some of these disadvantages. The number of injection ports has been doubled (from four to eight), and have been positioned more distally on the catheters' shaft resulting in a larger and more uniform zone of freezing on the balloons' surface [24] (**Figure 3**). The improved thermodynamic characteristics of the second-generation cryoballoon lead to a higher rate of single shot-PVI and a better chronic lesion durability. This high rate of durable PV isolation is anticipated to translate to improved clinical outcome [25].

Second-generation cryoballoon was found to be non-inferior to radiofrequency ablation in the FIRE and ICE randomized trial with respect to efficacy for the

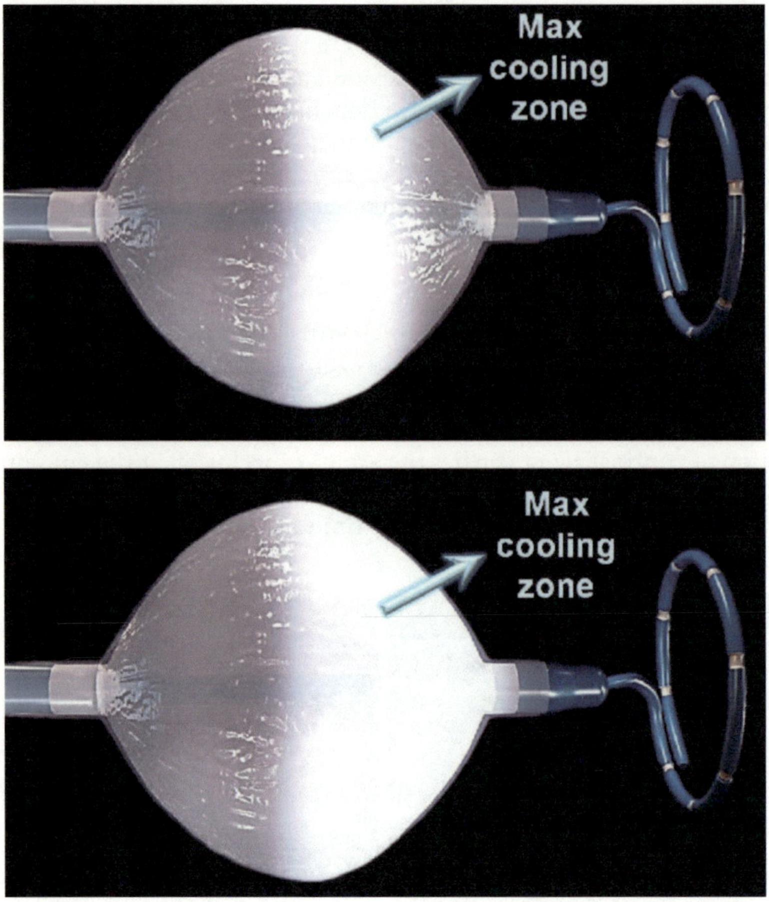

Figure 3.
First (upper part) and second (lower part) generation cryoballoons. First-generation cryoballoon produces an annular freezing zone at the balloon's equator. Second-generation cryoballoon has broader and more homogenous freezing zone, thus providing freezing at the whole distal hemisphere of the balloon.

treatment of patients with drug-refractory paroxysmal atrial fibrillation. There was also no significant difference between the two methods with regard to overall safety. Phrenic nerve injury was the most common safety event in the cryoballoon group [26]. The enlarged volume of tissue freezing may cause a trend toward higher incidence of phrenic nerve palsy in the case of the second-generation cryoballoons. However, these events are transient in most of the cases [27, 28].

A growing evidence suggests that second-generation cryoballoon is also safe and effective in patients with persistent AF [29, 30]. In persistent AF the isolation of the left atrial appendage as an adjunct to PVI may improve 1-year outcomes compared with the PVI-only strategy using cryoballoon [31].

However, the cryoballoon may be less effective in some anatomical variations of the pulmonary veins such as long left common trunk, additional pulmonary veins, or in the case of a more oval PV orifice [32, 33]. In some cases the complication rates may also differ in pulmonary venous anatomical variations [34].

2.2.2 Radiofrequency point-by-point ablation

Circumferential pulmonary vein isolation with radiofrequency ablation was the first type of ablation that was proven to be superior compared with the antiarrhythmic drug treatment [35]. It requires limited use of fluoroscopy, because catheter guidance is achieved with the use of an electroanatomical mapping system. The disadvantage of the technology is that the approach requires extensive training due to the need for a more accurate catheter manipulation. It is both proven to be effective in paroxysmal and persistent AF in terms of reducing symptoms related to AF [36, 37]. Moreover it may have a positive effect on mortality in heart failure patients [38–40].

2.2.2.1 Radiofrequency point-by-point ablation with contact force-sensing catheters

The clinical efficacy of catheter ablation of AF remained limited by difficulty in achieving durable pulmonary vein isolation. Suboptimal catheter tip-to-tissue contact force (CF) during lesion delivery may result in a reduced clinical efficacy. Despite the fact that acute PVI is nearly universally achieved, recurrences of atrial arrhythmias after AF ablation are common, and recurrences are usually due to PV reconnection and indicate insufficient lesion formation during the initial ablation.

A few years ago, contact force-sensing ablation catheters (CFSAC) have been introduced in the clinical practice. It has been shown that the contact force between the catheter tip and the target tissue is a key factor to a safe and effective lesion formation. Insufficient CF may result in an ineffective lesion, whereas excessive CF may result in complications such as heart wall perforation, steam pop, thrombus formation, or esophageal injury. High CF values may occur during catheter manipulation and not just during ablation, suggesting that measuring CF may provide additional useful information to the operator for safe catheter manipulation.

Catheter ablation using real-time CF technology was shown to be safe for the treatment of supraventricular tachycardias and AF [5, 6]. Pulmonary vein isolation with the use of contact force information results in a shorter procedure duration and a lower rate of AF recurrence after 12 months than conventional PVI without this information [41]. Analysis of the first trials with CFSACs showed that CF during catheter ablation for AF correlates with clinical outcome. Arrhythmia control is best achieved when ablation lesions are placed with an average CF of >20 g, whereas clinical failure is noted with an average CF of <10 g [8, 42].

The EFFICAS I multicenter study was to demonstrate the correlation between CF parameters during initial procedure and the incidence of isolation gaps at a repeated left atrial procedure at 3 months. To characterize the effect of CF applied over time, the system automatically detects the beginning and end of RF current delivery and calculates the force-time integral (FTI) defined as the total CF integrated over the time of RF delivery. Ablations with minimum FTI <400 g showed increased likelihood for reconnection. Thus, optimal CF parameter recommendations became a target CF of 20 g and a minimum FTI of 400 g for each lesion [7]. These recommendations together with contiguous lesion deployment were then confirmed by the EFFICAS II study as procedures with the abovementioned criteria resulted in more durable PVI [4].

2.2.2.2 Radiofrequency point-by-point ablation guided by ablation index

The routine use of CFSACs improved the arrhythmia-free survival after PVI; however, the recurrence rate remained substantial.

Ablation index (AI) incorporates CF, power, and time in a weighted formula and predicts lesion depth. It works together with SmartTouch catheter and CARTO system (**Figures 4** and 5).

$$\text{Ablation Index} = \left(K * \int_0^t CF^a(\tau) P^b(\tau) d\tau \right)^c$$

Figure 4.
Mathematical formula for the ablation index.

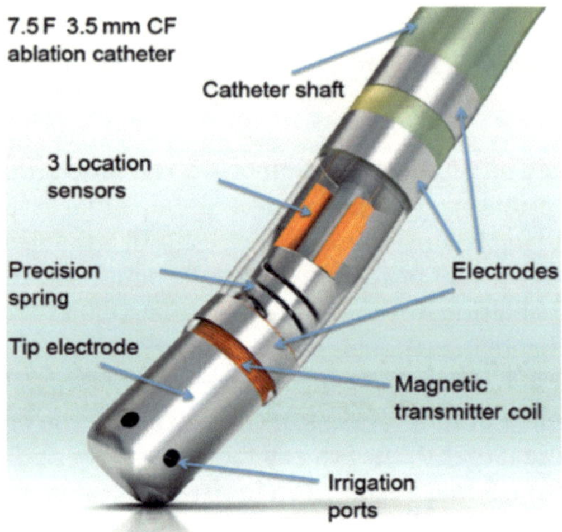

Figure 5.
SmartTouch catheter. This is a 7.5 French, 3.5-mm-irrigated-tip ablation catheter. Catheter tip contact force information and direction is measured by three location sensors within the shaft and the degree of spring bending via a magnetic transmitter at the catheter tip. The catheter and information are integrated into the Carto® 3 mapping system and can be displayed to the operators.

The analysis of PVIs guided by AI resulted in the development of the "CLOSE protocol." The CLOSE protocol is a new approach aiming to enclose the PVs with contiguous and optimized radiofrequency lesions by targeting an inter-lesion distance (ILD) ≤6 mm and AI ≥400 at the posterior wall and ≥550 at the anterior wall [11]. In the case of chest pain or intraesophageal temperature rise >38.5°C during posterior wall ablation, energy delivery may be stopped at an AI of 300. Target AI values can be reached with higher-energy applications as well (**Figures 6** and 7).

The use of CLOSE protocol was associated with high incidence of first-pass isolation (98%). Overall, single-procedure arrhythmia-free survival was 91% at 1 year without antiarrhythmic drug treatment. These findings are in line with the hypothesis that avoiding weak links within the deployed radiofrequency circle is the key to durable PVI and clinical success. These procedural results do not compromise safety and are associated with relatively short procedure and ablation times [12].

The optimal AI target values are not determined yet, and values recommended by the CLOSE protocol may overshoot. Lee et al. presented that PVIs with AI target values of ≥450 at the anterior/roof segments and of ≥350 at the posterior/inferior/carina segments are optimal AI thresholds for avoiding acute pulmonary vein reconnection [9]. In the left atrium, the AI-impedance relationship plateaus from 430 AI for the SmartTouch catheter, suggesting ablation beyond this value, have minimal additional biophysical benefit [43]. Solimene et al. found that radiofrequency energy targeting inter-lesion distance ≤6 mm and ablation index of 330–350 at posterior wall and 400–450 at anterior wall produces similar good results and low complication rates [44]. Another study found that no reconnection was seen where the minimum AI value was ≥370 for posterior/inferior segments and ≥480 for anterior/roof segments at repeat electrophysiology study [45].

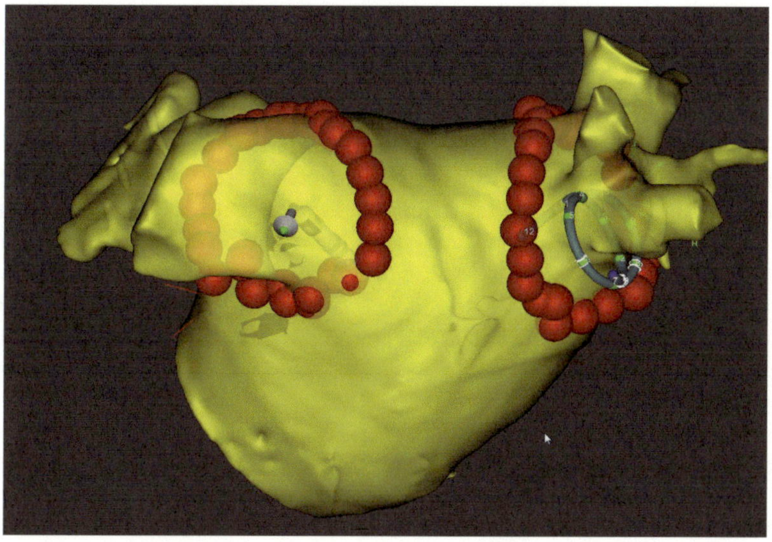

Figure 6.
Pulmonary vein isolation (CT-merged CARTO image) performed with CLOSE protocol. Red ablation tags indicate AI value >400 on the posterior wall and >550 on the anterior wall.

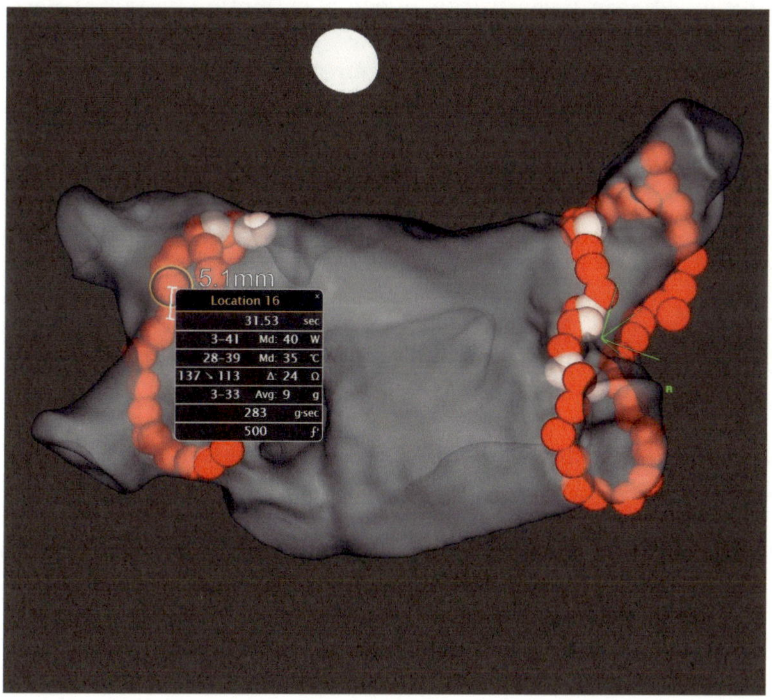

Figure 7.
Pulmonary vein isolation (CARTO, fast anatomical map) performed with CLOSE protocol. Ablation parameters of the highlighted dot (with yellow ring around it) are shown, including application duration, power, temperature, impedance drop, average contact force, force-time integral value, and ablation index value (AI = 500 in this case). The inter-lesion distance between the two marked ablation points (with distance measurement white line between them) is also shown (ILD = 5.1 mm).

The use of AI and small ILD results in a high level of durable PVI and may be also effective in persistent AF. A good clinical outcome can be achieved in the great majority of patients with persistent AF [10].

2.2.2.3 Esophageal temperatures during applications with ablation index

The incidence of endoscopically detected esophageal injury after catheter ablation is high (2–30%), both after PVI guided by cryoballoon and by RF energy [46–49]. High AI target values may further increase the risk of esophageal lesions.

The incidence of esophageal injury on endoscopy after CLOSE-guided PVI is low (1.2%) despite significant intraesophageal temperature rise during the procedure [50]. The most likely explanation of the low incidence after CLOSE PVI is the ablation protocol itself as AI target value on posterior wall is recommended to be reduced to 300 if pain or esophageal temperature rise occurs. Moreover, the high incidence of first-pass isolation results in smaller amount of applications required to reach the complete PVI.

3. Ablation strategies in persistent atrial fibrillation

Persistent AF is usually a more difficult arrhythmia as compared with the paroxysmal AF. Besides the triggers that induce the arrhythmia, usually a complex substrate is also present due to the atrial enlargement and fibrosis. Thus, pulmonary vein isolation alone is generally less effective than in paroxysmal AF [51]. The success rate of catheter ablation might improve with substrate modification techniques such as additional linear lines, ablation of complex fractionated atrial electrograms, and isolation of the left atrial appendage. The value of these techniques is controversial; however, most of the studies that compared PVI to PVI plus substrate modification were performed before the contact force era and in low-volume centers [29, 31, 52–56]. Substrate modification of persistent AF with the ablation of additional lines may be useful if procedure is performed by experienced operators. Kettering et al. found better arrhythmia-free survival in patients with roofline ablation when added to PVI (72 vs. 63%) [57]. Additional mitral isthmus line ablation may also provide a higher success rate as shown by Jais et al. (87 vs. 69%) [58].

4. Our personal approach for atrial fibrillation ablation

Here we shortly summarize our personal approach for PVI that we use in the Electrophysiology Laboratory of the Heart and Vascular Center, Semmelweis University, Budapest.

In case of symptomatic paroxysmal atrial fibrillation, the primary goal is the durable isolation of all pulmonary veins. Before the procedure cardiac CT or MR angiography is performed to evaluate the presence of potential coronary artery disease and to determine the pulmonary venous anatomy. For patients with typical anatomy (four distinct pulmonary veins), we may choose cryoballoon; however, a vast majority of patients are ablated with point-by-point approach with contact force-sensing ablation catheters. For the latter we may use CARTO or EnSite navigation system. For repeated ablations we first check the pulmonary veins, and if there is reconnection, we re-isolate the PVs with CARTO, EnSite, or Rhythmia system. If all the pulmonary veins are found to be isolated, then we try to find and eliminate non-PV triggers such as superior vena cava or coronary sinus.

In the case of symptomatic persistent atrial fibrillation, the first procedure is also pulmonary vein isolation similar to the paroxysmal cases. For repeated ablations besides re-isolation of PVs, we may use additional ablation lines such as left atrial roofline, posterior line, mitral isthmus line, and in the right atrium the cavo-tricuspidal isthmus line. If the recurrent arrhythmia is a macro-reentrant atrial tachycardia, we perform an electroanatomical activation map to depict the tachycardia circuit and to find the optimal ablation target(s).

5. Conclusion

Pulmonary vein isolation (PVI) is the cornerstone of rhythm-control therapy for atrial fibrillation (AF). A few years ago, new technologies such as cryoballoon and contact force-sensing ablation catheters were introduced. The use of these technologies became the part of the everyday practice. The routine use of CF ablation catheters and cryoballoons improved the arrhythmia-free survival after PVI; however, the recurrence rate remained substantial. The durability of PVI depends much on the accurate lesion creation. The recently developed techniques such as second-generation cryoballoon, ablation index, and CLOSE protocol may result in a higher rate of both acute PVI and thus a more durable lesion creation. The CLOSE protocol is a new approach aiming to enclose the PVs with contiguous and optimized radiofrequency lesions. This high rate of durable PV isolation is anticipated to translate to improved clinical outcome for both paroxysmal and persistent atrial fibrillation. Substrate modification of persistent AF with the ablation of additional lines may be useful if procedure is performed by experienced operators.

Conflict of interest

The authors declare no conflict of interest.

Author details

Nándor Szegedi and László Gellér*
Heart and Vascular Center, Semmelweis University, Budapest, Hungary

*Address all correspondence to: laszlo.geller@gmail.com

References

[1] Benjamin EJ, Wolf PA, D'Agostino RB, Silbershatz H, Kannel WB, Levy D. Impact of atrial fibrillation on the risk of death: The Framingham heart study. Circulation. 1998;**98**(10):946-952

[2] Kirchhof P, Benussi S, Kotecha D, Ahlsson A, Atar D, Casadei B, et al. ESC guidelines for the management of atrial fibrillation developed in collaboration with EACTS. European Heart Journal. 2016;**37**(38):2893-2962

[3] Packer DL, Mark DB, Robb RA, Monahan KH, Bahnson TD, Poole JE, et al. Effect of catheter ablation vs antiarrhythmic drug therapy on mortality, stroke, bleeding, and cardiac arrest among patients with atrial fibrillation: The CABANA randomized clinical trial. JAMA. 2019;**321**(13):1261-1274

[4] Kautzner J, Neuzil P, Lambert H, Peichl P, Petru J, Cihak R, et al. EFFICAS II: Optimization of catheter contact force improves outcome of pulmonary vein isolation for paroxysmal atrial fibrillation. Europace. 2015;**17**(8):1229-1235

[5] Kuck KH, Reddy VY, Schmidt B, Natale A, Neuzil P, Saoudi N, et al. A novel radiofrequency ablation catheter using contact force sensing: Toccata study. Heart Rhythm. 2012;**9**(1):18-23

[6] Natale A, Reddy VY, Monir G, Wilber DJ, Lindsay BD, McElderry HT, et al. Paroxysmal AF catheter ablation with a contact force sensing catheter: Results of the prospective, multicenter SMART-AF trial. Journal of the American College of Cardiology. 2014;**64**(7):647-656

[7] Neuzil P, Reddy VY, Kautzner J, Petru J, Wichterle D, Shah D, et al. Electrical reconnection after pulmonary vein isolation is contingent on contact force during initial treatment: Results from the EFFICAS I study. Circulation: Arrhythmia and Electrophysiology. 2013;**6**(2):327-333

[8] Reddy VY, Dukkipati SR, Neuzil P, Natale A, Albenque JP, Kautzner J, et al. Randomized, controlled trial of the safety and effectiveness of a contact force-sensing irrigated catheter for ablation of paroxysmal atrial fibrillation: Results of the TactiCath contact force ablation catheter study for atrial fibrillation (TOCCASTAR) study. Circulation. 2015;**132**(10):907-915

[9] Lee SR, Choi EK, Lee EJ, Choe WS, Cha MJ, Oh S. Efficacy of the optimal ablation index-targeted strategy for pulmonary vein isolation in patients with atrial fibrillation: The OPTIMUM study results. Journal of Interventional Cardiac Electrophysiology. Aug 2019;**55**(2):171-181

[10] Hussein A, Das M, Riva S, Morgan M, Ronayne C, Sahni A, et al. Use of ablation index-guided ablation results in high rates of durable pulmonary vein isolation and freedom from arrhythmia in persistent atrial fibrillation patients. Circulation: Arrhythmia and Electrophysiology. 2018;**11**(9):e006576

[11] Phlips T, Taghji P, El Haddad M, Wolf M, Knecht S, Vandekerckhove Y, et al. Improving procedural and one-year outcome after contact force-guided pulmonary vein isolation: The role of interlesion distance, ablation index, and contact force variability in the 'CLOSE'-protocol. Europace. 2018;**20**(FI_3):f419-f427

[12] Taghji P, El Haddad M, Phlips T, Wolf M, Knecht S, Vandekerckhove Y, et al. Evaluation of a strategy aiming to enclose the pulmonary veins with

contiguous and optimized radiofrequency lesions in paroxysmal atrial fibrillation: A pilot study. JACC: Clinical Electrophysiology. 2018;**4**(1):99-108

[13] Haissaguerre M, Jais P, Shah DC, Takahashi A, Hocini M, Quiniou G, et al. Spontaneous initiation of atrial fibrillation by ectopic beats originating in the pulmonary veins. The New England Journal of Medicine. 1998;**339**(10):659-666

[14] Jais P, Hocini M, Macle L, Choi KJ, Deisenhofer I, Weerasooriya R, et al. Distinctive electrophysiological properties of pulmonary veins in patients with atrial fibrillation. Circulation. 2002;**106**(19):2479-2485

[15] Rostock T, Steven D, Lutomsky B, Servatius H, Drewitz I, Klemm H, et al. Atrial fibrillation begets atrial fibrillation in the pulmonary veins on the impact of atrial fibrillation on the electrophysiological properties of the pulmonary veins in humans. Journal of the American College of Cardiology. 2008;**51**(22):2153-2160

[16] Knight BP. The pulmonary veins speedy recoveries and early discharges. Journal of the American College of Cardiology. 2008;**51**(22):2161-2162

[17] De Ponti R, Tritto M, Lanzotti ME, Spadacini G, Marazzi R, Moretti P, et al. Computerized high-density mapping of the pulmonary veins: New insights into their electrical activation in patients with atrial fibrillation. Europace. 2004;**6**(2):97-108

[18] Pappone C, Santinelli V, Manguso F, Vicedomini G, Gugliotta F, Augello G, et al. Pulmonary vein denervation enhances long-term benefit after circumferential ablation for paroxysmal atrial fibrillation. Circulation. 2004;**109**(3):327-334

[19] Mandapati R, Skanes A, Chen J, Berenfeld O, Jalife J. Stable microreentrant sources as a mechanism of atrial fibrillation in the isolated sheep heart. Circulation. 2000;**101**(2):194-199

[20] Hwang C, Wu TJ, Doshi RN, Peter CT, Chen PS. Vein of Marshall cannulation for the analysis of electrical activity in patients with focal atrial fibrillation. Circulation. 2000;**101**(13):1503-1505

[21] Sueda T, Nagata H, Orihashi K, Morita S, Okada K, Sueshiro M, et al. Efficacy of a simple left atrial procedure for chronic atrial fibrillation in mitral valve operations. The Annals of Thoracic Surgery. 1997;**63**(4):1070-1075

[22] Yorgun H, Aytemir K, Canpolat U, Sahiner L, Kaya EB, Oto A. Additional benefit of cryoballoon-based atrial fibrillation ablation beyond pulmonary vein isolation: Modification of ganglionated plexi. Europace. 2014;**16**(5):645-651

[23] Luik A, Radzewitz A, Kieser M, Walter M, Bramlage P, Hormann P, et al. Cryoballoon versus open irrigated radiofrequency ablation in patients with paroxysmal atrial fibrillation: The prospective, randomized, controlled, noninferiority freeze AF study. Circulation. 2015;**132**(14):1311-1319

[24] Chierchia GB, Di Giovanni G, Ciconte G, de Asmundis C, Conte G, Sieira-Moret J, et al. Second-generation cryoballoon ablation for paroxysmal atrial fibrillation: 1-year follow-up. Europace. 2014;**16**(5):639-644

[25] Reddy VY, Sediva L, Petru J, Skoda J, Chovanec M, Chitovova Z, et al. Durability of pulmonary vein isolation with cryoballoon ablation: Results from the sustained PV isolation with arctic front advance (SUPIR) study. Journal of Cardiovascular Electrophysiology. 2015;**26**(5):493-500

[26] Kuck KH, Brugada J, Furnkranz A, Metzner A, Ouyang F, Chun KR, et al. Cryoballoon or radiofrequency ablation for paroxysmal atrial fibrillation. The New England Journal of Medicine. 2016;**374**(23):2235-2245

[27] Casado-Arroyo R, Chierchia GB, Conte G, Levinstein M, Sieira J, Rodriguez-Manero M, et al. Phrenic nerve paralysis during cryoballoon ablation for atrial fibrillation: A comparison between the first- and second-generation balloon. Heart Rhythm. 2013;**10**(9):1318-1324

[28] Furnkranz A, Bordignon S, Schmidt B, Perrotta L, Dugo D, De Lazzari M, et al. Incidence and characteristics of phrenic nerve palsy following pulmonary vein isolation with the second-generation as compared with the first-generation cryoballoon in 360 consecutive patients. Europace. 2015;**17**(4):574-578

[29] Omran H, Gutleben KJ, Molatta S, Fischbach T, Wellmann B, Horstkotte D, et al. Second generation cryoballoon ablation for persistent atrial fibrillation: An updated meta-analysis. Clinical Research in Cardiology. 2018;**107**(2):182-192

[30] Canpolat U, Kocyigit D, Yalcin MU, Coteli C, Sener YZ, Oksul M, et al. Long-term outcomes of pulmonary vein isolation using second-generation cryoballoon during atrial fibrillation ablation. Pacing and Clinical Electrophysiology. Jul 2019;**42**(7):910-921

[31] Yorgun H, Canpolat U, Kocyigit D, Coteli C, Evranos B, Aytemir K. Left atrial appendage isolation in addition to pulmonary vein isolation in persistent atrial fibrillation: One-year clinical outcome after cryoballoon-based ablation. Europace. 2017;**19**(5):758-768

[32] Yalin K, Lyan E, Abdin A, Heeger CH, Vogler J, Liosis S, et al. Second-generation cryoballoon for pulmonary vein isolation in patients with pulmonary vein abnormality: Safety, efficacy and lessons from re-ablation procedures. International Journal of Cardiology. 2018;**272**:142-148

[33] Shigeta T, Okishige K, Yamauchi Y, Aoyagi H, Nakamura T, Yamashita M, et al. Clinical assessment of cryoballoon ablation in cases with atrial fibrillation and a left common pulmonary vein. Journal of Cardiovascular Electrophysiology. 2017;**28**(9):1021-1027

[34] Stroker E, de Asmundis C, Saitoh Y, Velagic V, Mugnai G, Irfan G, et al. Anatomic predictors of phrenic nerve injury in the setting of pulmonary vein isolation using the 28-mm second-generation cryoballoon. Heart Rhythm. 2016;**13**(2):342-351

[35] Pappone C, Vicedomini G, Augello G, Manguso F, Saviano M, Baldi M, et al. Radiofrequency catheter ablation and antiarrhythmic drug therapy: A prospective, randomized, 4-year follow-up trial: The APAF study. Circulation: Arrhythmia and Electrophysiology. 2011;**4**(6):808-814

[36] Chen J, Dagres N, Hocini M, Fauchier L, Bongiorni MG, Defaye P, et al. Catheter ablation for atrial fibrillation: Results from the first European snapshot survey on procedural routines for atrial fibrillation ablation (ESS-PRAFA). Part II. Europace. 2015;**17**(11):1727-1732

[37] Nielsen JC, Johannessen A, Raatikainen P, Hindricks G, Walfridsson H, Pehrson SM, et al. Long-term efficacy of catheter ablation as first-line therapy for paroxysmal atrial fibrillation: 5-year outcome in a randomised clinical trial. Heart. 2017;**103**(5):368-376

[38] Hunter RJ, Berriman TJ, Diab I, Kamdar R, Richmond L, Baker V, et al. A randomized controlled trial of

catheter ablation versus medical treatment of atrial fibrillation in heart failure (the CAMTAF trial). Circulation: Arrhythmia and Electrophysiology. 2014;**7**(1):31-38

[39] Marrouche NF, Brachmann J, Andresen D, Siebels J, Boersma L, Jordaens L, et al. Catheter ablation for atrial fibrillation with heart failure. The New England Journal of Medicine. 2018;**378**(5):417-427

[40] Di Biase L, Mohanty P, Mohanty S, Santangeli P, Trivedi C, Lakkireddy D, et al. Ablation versus amiodarone for treatment of persistent atrial fibrillation in patients with congestive heart failure and an implanted device: Results from the AATAC multicenter randomized trial. Circulation. 2016;**133**(17):1637-1644

[41] Wutzler A, Huemer M, Parwani AS, Blaschke F, Haverkamp W, Boldt LH. Contact force mapping during catheter ablation for atrial fibrillation: Procedural data and one-year follow-up. Archives of Medical Science. 2014;**10**(2):266-272

[42] Reddy VY, Shah D, Kautzner J, Schmidt B, Saoudi N, Herrera C, et al. The relationship between contact force and clinical outcome during radiofrequency catheter ablation of atrial fibrillation in the TOCCATA study. Heart Rhythm. 2012;**9**(11):1789-1795

[43] Ullah W, Hunter RJ, Finlay MC, McLean A, Dhinoja MB, Sporton S, et al. Ablation index and surround flow catheter irrigation: Impedance-based appraisal in clinical ablation. JACC: Clinical Electrophysiology. 2017;**3**(10):1080-1088

[44] Solimene F, Schillaci V, Shopova G, Urraro F, Arestia A, Iuliano A, et al. Safety and efficacy of atrial fibrillation ablation guided by ablation index module. Journal of Interventional Cardiac Electrophysiology. 2019;**54**(1):9-15

[45] Das M, Loveday JJ, Wynn GJ, Gomes S, Saeed Y, Bonnett LJ, et al. Ablation index, a novel marker of ablation lesion quality: Prediction of pulmonary vein reconnection at repeat electrophysiology study and regional differences in target values. Europace. 2017;**19**(5):775-783

[46] Yarlagadda B, Deneke T, Turagam M, Dar T, Paleti S, Parikh V, et al. Temporal relationships between esophageal injury type and progression in patients undergoing atrial fibrillation catheter ablation. Heart Rhythm. 2019;**16**(2):204-212

[47] Martinek M, Meyer C, Hassanein S, Aichinger J, Bencsik G, Schoefl R, et al. Identification of a high-risk population for esophageal injury during radiofrequency catheter ablation of atrial fibrillation: Procedural and anatomical considerations. Heart Rhythm. 2010;**7**(9):1224-1230

[48] Blockhaus C, Muller P, Vom Dahl S, Leonhardt S, Haussinger D, Gerguri S, et al. Low incidence of esophageal lesions after pulmonary vein isolation using contact-force sensing catheter without esophageal temperature probe. International Heart Journal. 2017;**58**(6):880-884

[49] Muller P, Dietrich JW, Halbfass P, Abouarab A, Fochler F, Szollosi A, et al. Higher incidence of esophageal lesions after ablation of atrial fibrillation related to the use of esophageal temperature probes. Heart Rhythm. 2015;**12**(7):1464-1469

[50] Wolf M, El Haddad M, De Wilde V, Phlips T, De Pooter J, Almorad A, et al. Endoscopic evaluation of the esophagus after catheter ablation of atrial fibrillation using contiguous and optimized radiofrequency applications. Heart Rhythm. Jul 2019;**16**(7):1013-1020

[51] Schreiber D, Rostock T, Frohlich M, Sultan A, Servatius H, Hoffmann BA, et al. Five-year follow-up after catheter ablation of persistent atrial fibrillation using the stepwise approach and prognostic factors for success. Circulation: Arrhythmia and Electrophysiology. 2015;**8**(2):308-317

[52] Verma A, Jiang CY, Betts TR, Chen J, Deisenhofer I, Mantovan R, et al. Approaches to catheter ablation for persistent atrial fibrillation. The New England Journal of Medicine. 2015;**372**(19):1812-1822

[53] Verma A, Mantovan R, Macle L, De Martino G, Chen J, Morillo CA, et al. Substrate and trigger ablation for reduction of atrial fibrillation (STAR AF): A randomized, multicentre, international trial. European Heart Journal. 2010;**31**(11):1344-1356

[54] Friedman DJ, Black-Maier EW, Barnett AS, Pokorney SD, Al-Khatib SM, Jackson KP, et al. Left atrial appendage electrical isolation for treatment of recurrent atrial fibrillation: A meta-analysis. JACC: Clinical Electrophysiology. 2018;**4**(1):112-120

[55] Di Biase L, Burkhardt JD, Mohanty P, Mohanty S, Sanchez JE, Trivedi C, et al. Left atrial appendage isolation in patients with longstanding persistent AF undergoing catheter ablation: BELIEF trial. Journal of the American College of Cardiology. 2016;**68**(18):1929-1940

[56] Fink T, Schluter M, Heeger CH, Lemes C, Maurer T, Reissmann B, et al. Stand-alone pulmonary vein isolation versus pulmonary vein isolation with additional substrate modification as index ablation procedures in patients with persistent and long-standing persistent atrial fibrillation: The randomized alster-lost-AF trial (ablation at St. Georg Hospital for Long-Standing Persistent Atrial Fibrillation). Circulation: Arrhythmia and Electrophysiology. 2017;**10**:e005114

[57] Kettering K, Yim DH, Gramley F. Catheter ablation of persistent atrial fibrillation: Circumferential pulmonary vein ablation: Beneficial effect of an additional linear lesion at the roof of the left atrium on the long-term outcome. Herzschrittmachertherapie & Elektrophysiologie. 2017;**28**(3):328-334

[58] Jais P, Hocini M, Hsu LF, Sanders P, Scavee C, Weerasooriya R, et al. Technique and results of linear ablation at the mitral isthmus. Circulation. 2004;**110**(19):2996-3002

Chapter 6

Surgical Treatment of Atrial Fibrillation

Manoraj Navaratnarajah, Suvitesh Luthra and Sunil Ohri

Abstract

The concepts, techniques and evidence relating to surgical ablation of atrial fibrillation are discussed in detail. The historical background to surgical ablation is covered in brief, along with the electrophysiological basis underpinning its effective useage. The epidemiology of surgically treated atrial fibrillation and the current guidelines relating to its use are analysed. Safety aspects and perspectives on its ongoing future use are discussed. Modern surgical technologies and approaches are reviewed, along with the relevant advantages and disadvantages of each. The surgical techniques relating to left atrial appendage intervention are also reviewed, along with the relevant literature and evidence relating to reduction in thromboembolic risk and need for anticoagulation.

Keywords: MAZE, left trial appendage, surgical ablation

1. Epidemiology of atrial fibrillation

Atrial fibrillation (AF) is the most common type of cardiac arrhythmia and remains a major cause of stroke, heart failure (HF), sudden death, and cardiovascular morbidity. Importantly, with an ever-ageing population, the prevalence of AF is increasing, and predicted to rise steeply in the future [1]. AF impairs functional status, cognitive function and reduces the quality of life [2]. Age, sex, race, and geographical location, as well as other modifiable risk factors (diabetes, hypertension, lung disease, obesity and alcohol use) determine the prevalence of AF. The overall prevalence of AF is approximately 1%, but rises significantly with age. In those over 75 years old it has been shown to be greater than 10%, and greater than 15% in those over 85 [3, 4].

As such, the proportion of patients presenting for cardiac surgery in AF, or with a history of AF is also expanding. AF detrimentally affects prognosis in patients with severe valvular heart disease [5], and those undergoing surgery or transcatheter interventions for aortic or mitral valve disease, and in combination with valvular heart disease, increases thromboembolic risk significantly [6, 7]. As with congestive HF, valvular disease and AF share a dynamic interaction that sustain one another, driven by the detrimental effects of volume and pressure overload, maladaptive neurohumoral activation, cardiac fibrosis and a deleterious tachy-cardiomyopathy. Therefore, it is intuitive that immense attention has been, and continues to be focussed upon the potential likely benefits of surgical correction of AF, as part of both concomitant AND stand-alone procedures.

1.1 Atrial fibrillation in surgical patients

The prevalence of pre-operative AF varies with the encountered cardiac pathology, and this, together with surgical procedure type, influences the likelihood of concomitant surgical AF ablation. In the surgical population, the prevalence is greatly skewed towards mitral valve disease, because this pathology invokes the greatest degree of left atrial (LA) distension [8]. An AF prevalence of 30% is reported in mitral valve surgical patients, and only 14% and 6% in patients undergoing aortic valve or isolated coronary surgery, respectively [9]. Analysis of US registry data from the early 2000s showed that the prospect of concomitant AF ablation was greatest in mitral valve patients (~60%) and double that in aortic valve (~30%) and coronary artery bypass (~25%) surgical patients [10]. The chapter will focus upon the anatomical and physiological principles underlying surgical AF ablation, the technical and surgical aspects regarding specific anatomical lesion sets and their complications. Current evidence and guidelines supporting the use of surgical AF ablation, during both concomitant cardiac surgery and stand-alone surgery will also be reviewed.

2. Principles underlying surgical treatment of atrial fibrillation

A large variety of surgical strategies have evolved over past decades for the treatment of AF. As such, standardisation of terminology is difficult and comparison of studies can prove impossible. Anti-arrhythmic procedures are divided into two broad categories: (A) isolation or (B) ablation procedures. Initial surgical procedures were isolation procedures, aimed at confining the arrhythmia to a specific region of the heart [11]. Ablation was not carried out at this early time, as there was insufficient knowledge relating to the electrophysiological mechanisms driving AF. Isolation procedures such as LA isolation and the corridor operation will not be reviewed further in this chapter as they are irrelevant to current clinical practice.

Starting in the 1980s, several procedures were developed in an effort to treat AF, including LA isolation (A), corridor operation (B), and atrial transection (C) (**Figure 1**). The first attempt to surgically ablate AF was made via the atrial transection procedure in 1986 [12]. This procedure failed after 5 months in the 1 patient in which it was performed. Transection was based upon on the flawed belief that AF was caused by two macro-re-entrant circuits; one around the SVC and IVC orifices and one around the pulmonary veins and the orifice of the LA appendage (LAA). With improving knowledge of the mechanisms driving AF the MAZE procedure and pulmonary vein isolation (PVI) subsequently evolved, and formed the foundation of modern surgical treatment of AF. These two procedures form the main focus of this chapter.

2.1 The MAZE concept

The MAZE concept underlying the classical MAZE procedure is best encapsulated by the words of Dr James Cox—'The cardinal feature of a classical MAZE procedure includes lines of conduction block that preclude macro-re-entry anywhere in either atrium while leaving both atria capable of activation by a sinus-generated impulse. Components essential to achieving this include appropriate lesions in *both* atria, the absence of gaps that allow electrical activity to bypass an intended line of block, and the absence of alternate pathways by which impulses can reach the intended maze exit'. 'The maze has one entrance site, one exit site and one true route between the entrance and exit' [13] (**Figure 2**). It must be stressed that numerous surgical ablation strategies are now in existence that do *not* strictly

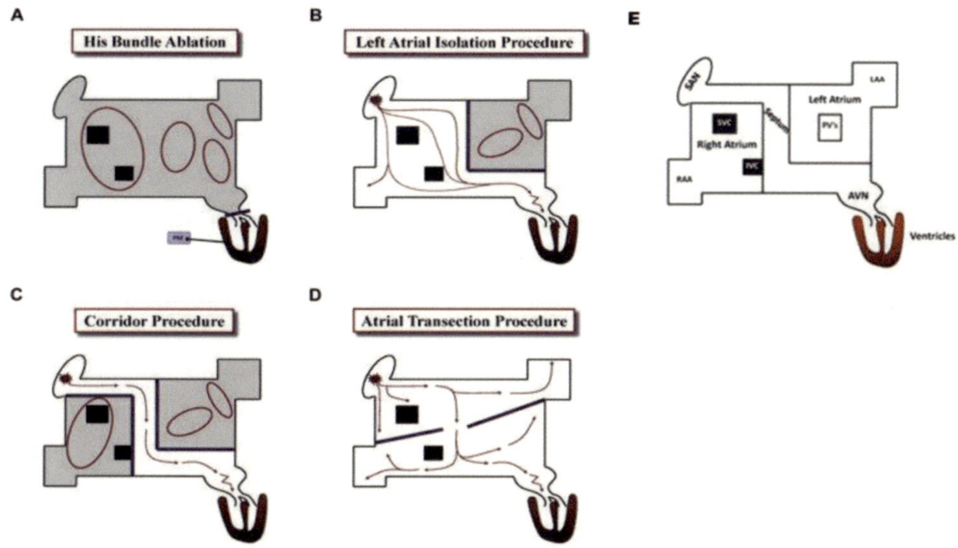

Figure 1.
Schematic representation of AF isolation/ablation techniques. (A) His bundle ablation, (B) Left atrial isolation procedure, (C) Corridor procedure (D) Atrial transection procedure and (E) MAZE concept [13].

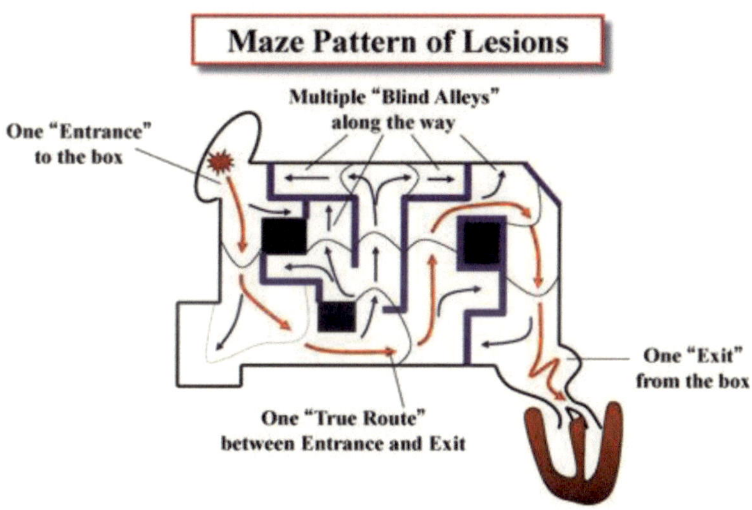

Figure 2.
Schematic representation of the surgical MAZE concept [13].

adhere to the MAZE concept described above, yet are described as 'MAZE' procedures. The implications of utilising this generic umbrella term, when comparing studies and drawing conclusions from study outcomes must be appreciated.

2.2 Surgical ablation lesion sets

The first MAZE-I procedure was performed in 1987. It abolished AF and re-established sinus rhythm (SR) effectively. However, the MAZE-I was associated with chronotropic incompetence in approximately 30% of patients, and intra-atrial conduction delay resulting in loss of LA transport due to simultaneous LA and left ventricle (LV) contraction [13]. These two undesirable effects of the MAZE-I procedure, led to modifications in the lesion set thus creating the MAZE

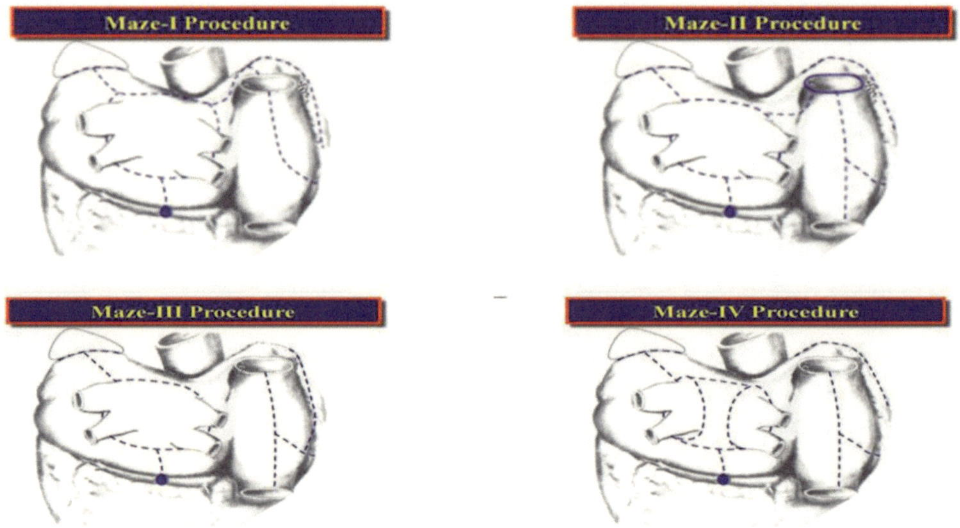

Figure 3.
Versions of the surgical MAZE procedure [13].

II procedure. The anterior-superior LA and right atrium (RA) lesions were repositioned in a more posterior location. The Maze II was performed in less than 15 patients, due to extreme technical difficulty that required SVC transection above the RA to enhance LA exposure [13, 14]. The MAZE III included relocation of anterior lesion sets further posteriorly and a septal lesion to facilitate LA exposure, the latter being omitted subsequently in later iterations of the MAZE III. From 1992 onwards the surgical cut-and sew MAZE-III procedure was performed through a median sternotomy, and the lesion pattern became the standard pattern for MAZE procedures. As the name implies, all cardiac lesions were created by cutting the full thickness of the myocardium and then re-sewing the tissue together, thus inhibiting macro re-entry circuit conduction. It was not until 1997 when the original cut-and-sew MAZE-III procedure was replaced by cryosurgical MAZE-III procedure, where all surgical lesions were replaced by cryoablation lesions created by a linear cryoprobe [13]. The MAZE III was then superseded by the first MAZE IV procedure in 2002. Lesion sets were essentially identical, with lesions in the MAZE IV performed using a combination of bipolar radiofrequency clamps and linear cryoprobes [15] (**Figure 3**). Improved speed of execution resulted in less patient morbidity during the MAZE IV, and this is now the gold standard procedure in AF ablation. Surgical AF ablation is most commonly applied as a concomitant procedure during valve or coronary revascularization operations, but also as a primary or stand-alone procedure. The frequency of surgical ablation and durable achievement of SR is increasing, represented mainly by the MAZE III/IV procedures.

3. Surgical ablation energy sources

Numerous energy sources have evolved over the past two decades to replace the traditional 'cut and sew' technique that aim to replicate transmural lesions, whilst enabling a less time-consuming yet equally effective approach. A fundamental pre-requisite for successful AF ablation, is complete transmurality and continuity bilaterally, and a correct lesion pattern.

3.1 Radiofrequency ablation

Radiofrequency ablation (RFA) acts by conducting an alternating electrical current through the myocardium. The energy of this electrical current disperses through myocardial tissue as heat, causing coagulative necrosis, creating an area of non-conducting myocardium. RFA employs an alternating current at 350 kHz-1 MHz to heat tissue to 70–80°C for 1 min, creating a 3–6 mm lesion using unipolar or bipolar devices. Transmurality is indicated by electrical conductance and impedance monitoring. The efficacy of AF ablation during cardiac surgery using either unipolar [16–18], or bipolar ablation [19–21] technology, is well established. Overall, success rates in restoring SR are over 60%, measured at a variety of time points ranging from 12 to 60 months post procedure. However, there is limited evidence to conclude whether bipolar RFA is more effective than unipolar RFA (**Figure 4**).

3.2 Cryoablation

Cryoablation works by using nitrous oxide as a cooling agent for 2 min at −60°C to produce a transmural lesion that can be visualised as an 'iceball'.

Tissue injury results by creation of ice crystals within cells disrupting the cell function and electrical conductivity. In addition, microvascular disruption causes cell death. Several studies have proven the efficacy of concomitant cryoablation in the treatment of AF. Cryoablation during concomitant cardiac surgery achieves good rates of SR, ranging from 60 to 80% at a variety of time points ranging from 12 to 60 months post procedure [22, 23] (**Figure 4**).

3.3 Microwave

Microwave ablation uses high-frequency electromagnetic radiation to induce oscillation of water molecules, and produces a well-demarcated lesion via thermal injury. Its main strength is the production of excellent epicardial lesions, thus promoting its use in minimally invasive techniques. A success rate ranging between 65 and 85% is observed over a variable follow up period between 6 and 12 months [24]. Long term success rates remain unclear and evidence relating to microwave ablation efficacy is limited. Thus far, bipolar RFA ablation and cryoablation have demonstrated superiority in terms of freedom from AF, AF recurrence rates, and microwave ablation is currently considered less effective than other ablation modalities [25, 26].

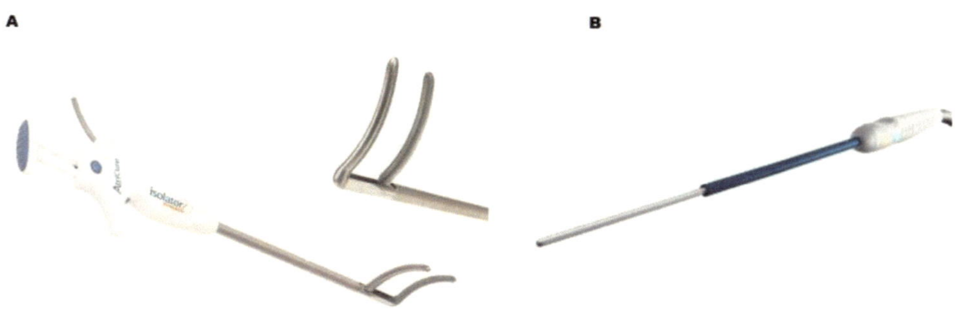

Figure 4.
Radiofrequency surgical ablation clamp (A) and cryoprobe (B) [105].

3.4 Laser and ultrasound

Alternative energy sources being explored in AF ablation are that of laser and ultrasound. Laser ablation uses a monochromatic, phase coherent beam to cause heating and cellular destruction. Laser has shown efficacy in restoration of SR (>70%) in isolated procedures and during concomitant surgery [27]. However, currently, laser ablation has not gained approval for clinical use outside of trials due to limited evidence supporting its efficacy and safety [27]. Ultrasound, utilises high-frequency sound waves (2–20 MHz) emitted by piezoelectric crystals to cause thermal heating and disruption of cell membranes. It creates permanent transmural lesions when applied epicardially and is advantageous in that CPB is unnecessary, and ablation can be executed on a beating heart. Ultrasound lesions can also be delivered via a balloon catheter, allowing isolated PVI [28, 29]. Reasonable conversion rates to SR have been demonstrated in isolated PVI for lone paroxysmal AF. However, due to frequent complications, such as atrio-oesophageal fistula, pericardial effusion and phrenic nerve palsy, use of ultrasound is not currently recommended, and its role in permanent AF is unproven [28, 29].

4. Surgical approaches for ablation

The MAZE IV can be performed either through a sternotomy or through a right mini thoracotomy. A combination of RFA and cryoablation is used to create the lesion set in the majority of cases. After gaining access to the chest both pulmonary veins are bluntly dissected, after initiating normothermic cardiopulmonary bypass (CPB). The patient is then cooled to 34°C and RA lesion set performed on a beating heart. A small purse-string suture at the base of the RA appendage allows one jaw of a RFA clamp to pass and create a lesion along the RA free wall (**Figure 5**). A vertical atriotomy extending from the intra-atrial septum up towards the atrioventricular

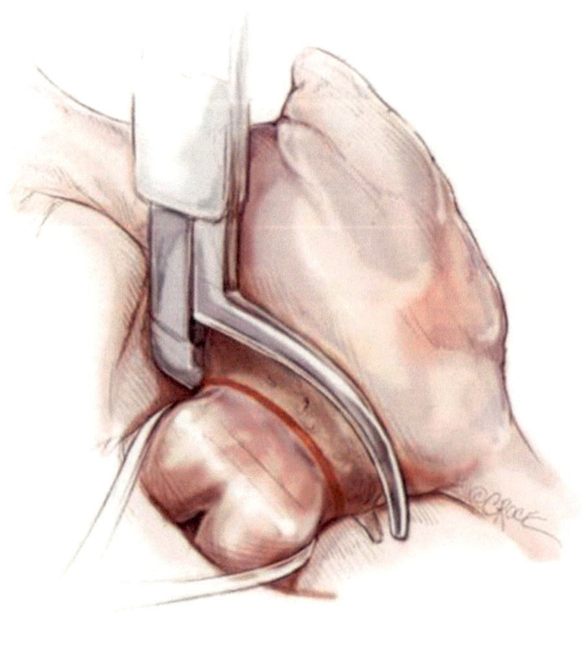

Figure 5.
Radiofrequency surgical ablation clamp performing right sided pulmonary vein isolation [106].

groove near the free margin of the heart is made at least 2 cm from the free wall lesion. From the inferior aspect of the incision, the RFA clamp then creates ablation lesions extending to the SVC and down towards the IVC. A linear cryoprobe is used to create an endocardial ablation on the tricuspid annulus at the two o'clock position. The cryoprobe is placed through the previously placed purse-string suture and an endocardial ablation is performed down to the 10 o'clock position on the tricuspid valve. When using a right mini-thoracotomy, the atriotomy is replaced by two additional purse-strings; one just above the intra-atrial septum midway between the SVC and IVC and one just next to the atrioventricular groove (**Figure 6**).

The LA lesion set is then performed under cardioplegic arrest. The LAA is amputated and the RFA clamp passed through to create a connecting lesion into the left superior pulmonary vein. The coronary sinus is marked with methylene blue at a point between the left and the right coronary arteries. A left atriotomy is performed and the posterior LA isolated using the RFA clamp both inferiorly and superiorly to connect the atriotomy to the previously made left pulmonary vein lesion (**Figure 7**). From the inferior part of the atriotomy an ablation lesion towards the mitral annulus is created. This lesion crosses the coronary sinus between the right coronary artery (RCA) and the circumflex artery. Cryoablation is then used to bridge the 2 cm gap from the end of the RFA lesion to the mitral valve annulus. Completion of the LA lesion set is carried out by cryoablating the coronary sinus in line with the isthmus lesion on the epicardial surface [30].

4.1 Thoracoscopic surgery

The MAZE IV is regarded as the gold standard surgical treatment for AF. However, the surgery although highly effective is quite invasive with related complications. Therefore, the totally thoracoscopic ablation procedure is gaining support as a minimally invasive alternative, and being performed both in a non-hybrid or (staged) hybrid setting. A large variety of thoracoscopic approaches are now established and regarded as safe [31] (**Figure 8**). Totally, thoracoscopic LA 'MAZE' procedures and PVI are described [32]. The procedures can be performed

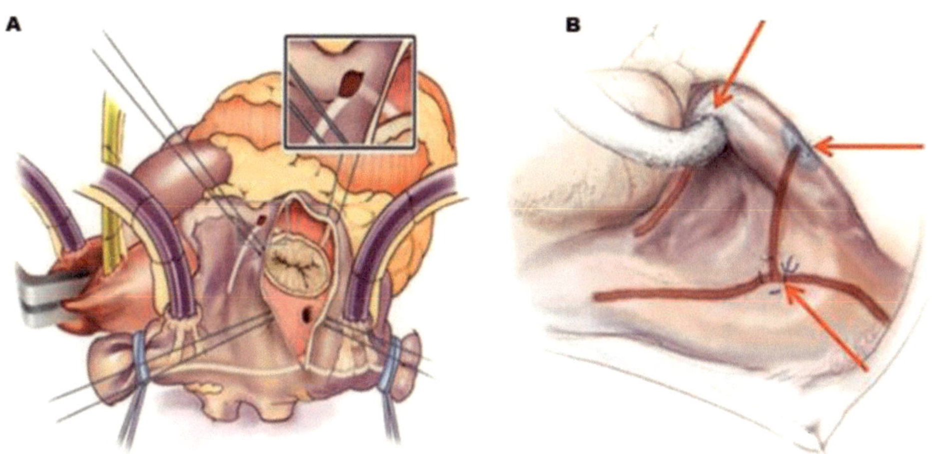

Figure 6.
Right atrial lesion sets for MAZE IV procedure. (A) Majority of linear lesions are created using bipolar radiofrequency clamps, and blue shades represent cryoablation lesions placed at two points on the tricuspid annulus through direct vision or small purse-string sutures (red arrows). (B) Linear lesions also can be created with cryoablation if required for mini-thoracotomy. Right atrial lesion set consisting of an ablation line along the SVC and IVC, ablation along the RA free wall with line to tricuspid valve annulus [106].

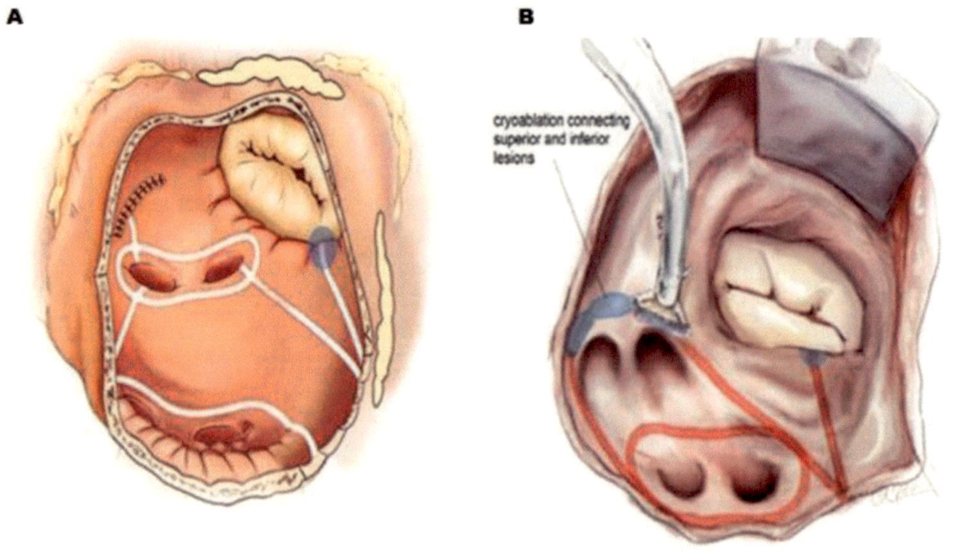

Figure 7.
Left atrial lesion sets for MAZE IV procedure. (A) Majority of linear lesions are created with bipolar radiofrequency clamps. Blue shades represent cryoablation lesions at the mitral isthmus and left pulmonary veins (minimally invasive approach). (B) Linear lesions can also be created with cryoablation if required for mini-thoracotomy. Left atrial lesion set consisting of bilateral PVI, pulmonary vein roof and floor connecting lesions, lesion from LSPV and amputated LAA, and lesion from inferior atriotomy to mitral valve annulus [106].

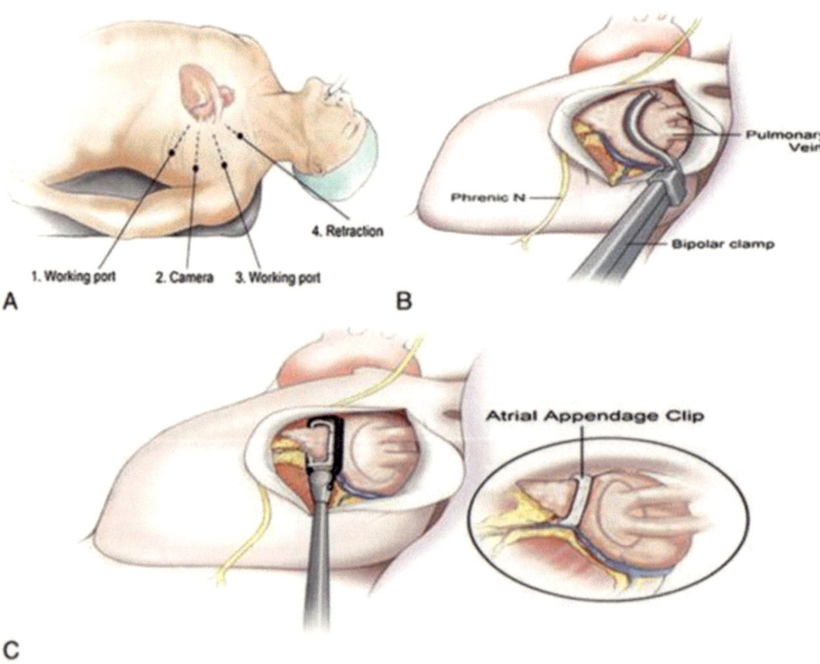

Figure 8.
Thoracoscopic PVI and LAA occlusion procedure. (A) Patient position and ports on left side. (B) Bipolar ablation clamp being placed around pulmonary vein hilum. (C) Clip being placed at the base of the left atrial appendage [107].

using three ports on both sides. On the right side, the pericardium is opened anterior to the phrenic nerve, followed by exploration of Waterston's groove for subsequent positioning of the ablation device. Prior to PVI, ganglionic plexus location is performed using a transpolar pen and high frequency pacing. A positive plexus location is ablated for 20 s with the transpolar pen. High-frequency pacing is again performed to confirm successful ganglionic plexus ablation, and repeated if necessary. After isolating the right pulmonary veins, some techniques include making a trigonum line. From the trigonum line, a separate lesion is made to the LAA. Blunt dissection around the PVs is performed using a dissector and PVI achieved by bipolar RFA ablation clamp. A minimum of three overlapping ablation lesions are performed at the antrum of the right PVs. Conduction block is confirmed, by the absence of PV potentials if AF is present; and by pacing if SR is present. Ablation is repeated if necessary. Both a roof line and a floor line are created with a linear pen, making up the box lesion. Left sided procedure is then carried out in a similar fashion; the pericardium is opened posterior to the phrenic nerve and ligament of Marshall divided. The LAAO is amputated/occluded by a verity of techniques [32, 33].

However, review of 14 thoracoscopic studies shows that a wide variety of lesion sets are used, most frequently the trigone line, connecting the roof line with the left fibrous trigone; the LAA line, connecting the superior PVs with the LAA; and the bi-caval line [31]. Most described techniques employ bipolar RFA.

4.2 COBRA Fusion device

There are many suitable types of minimally invasive ablation devices on the market and the box lesion technique is used in most of them. One such novel device is the COBRA Fusion device. For this device the transverse and oblique sinuses are bluntly dissected, along with the layer of fat in the area of the interatrial groove and transverse sinus. A special introducer, with a magnetic tip, is inserted into each sinus to meet behind the heart and form a loop, and the COBRA Fusion 150 (Estech, San Ramon, CA) ablation catheter is then connected to the introducer and pulled around the PVs (**Figure 9**).

Contact between atrial tissue and the catheter is then achieved using a unique suction device, with a target of suction of −500 mm Hg. The catheter uses unipolar and bipolar RFA to create lesions. The RFA is applied in 2 steps using temperature-control using a setting of 70°C for 60 s. Following this first cycle, the catheter is moved circumferentially to complete the box lesion and a second cycle of energy, both mono- and bipolar is applied. The continuity of lesion is checked visually in a reachable area, and a third overlapping ablation lesion performed if the line of the box lesion appears non-continuous. This third ablation is usually needed between the right superior pulmonary vein and the right inferior pulmonary vein mainly in patients with a large LA. In addition to visual inspection of the lesion line, in patients

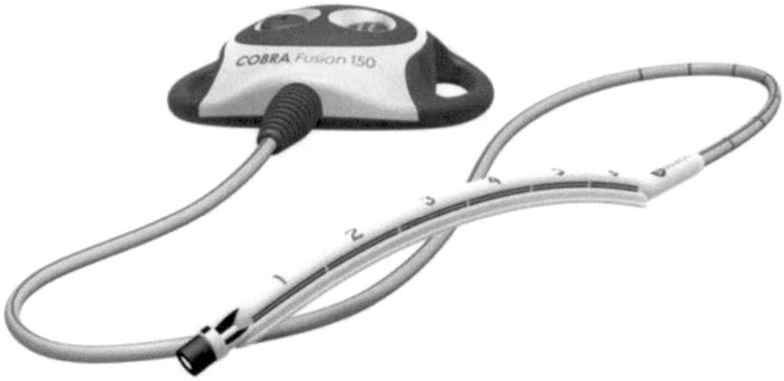

Figure 9.
COBRA Fusion surgical ablation device. A versatile and flexible design for epicardial ablation [105].

in SR exit block can be routinely tested by pacing the right PVs and the adjacent posterior LA, and another ablation performed if necessary. Of note however, successful box lesion isolation is only achievable in a minority of patients (<50%) [34].

5. Evidence and guidelines supporting surgical ablation

The majority of high-quality RCTs and meta-analyses of surgical ablation are weighted towards, but not confined to concomitant mitral procedures. As compared with patients in SR, those with AF tend to be older and to have worse baseline risk profiles. High baseline risk influences the decision not to perform concomitant ablation, nevertheless, the majority of studies advocate that worse risk profiles are not a contraindication to surgical ablation [35]. It is established that surgical ablation for AF can be performed without additional operative risk of mortality or major morbidity [35, 36]. Indeed, recent US registry data suggests that surgical ablation is associated with reduced mortality in multiple valve populations [37]. Currently, US guidelines recommended concomitant ablation during mitral surgery (Class 1, Level A), AVR, isolated CABG, and AVR + CABG (Class1, Level B) [35].

Surgical ablation for symptomatic AF in the absence of structural heart disease, refractory to medical therapy or catheter-based therapies, receives a class II recommendation as a primary stand-alone procedure (Level B). In addition, surgical ablation for symptomatic persistent or long-standing AF in the absence of structural heart disease is deemed reasonable as a stand-alone procedure, using the MAZE III/IV in comparison to PVI alone (Class IIA, Level B). Current literature shows that few technical restrictions are present opposing surgical ablation at the time of open atrial operations, and most studies agree that AF incidence is approximately halved, with this benefit maintained at 1 year [35, 37].

5.1 Safety and efficacy of surgical ablation

Clear direct demonstration of survival benefit following surgical ablation is not straight forward, due to heterogeneous study groups, follow-up periods and limited sample sizes. However, a clear link between restoration of SR and survival is verified in the literature. Regardless of survival benefit, long-term quality of life improvement following surgical ablation has been demonstrated by many, but not all studies [38, 39]. Surgical ablation does not abolish stroke risk, but has been associated with reduction in long-term stroke risk.

Surgically untreated AF correlates with increased morbidity and mortality following AVR [40], and freedom from AF is greater after concomitant surgical AF ablation [35]. Reluctance to open the atria during AVR and or CABG discourages full MAZE procedures, and less extensive/invasive epicardial ablative methods are often favoured. Therefore, the potential consequences of non-adherence to the strict MAZE principles outlined earlier, on outcomes must be appreciated. As such, SR recovery appears to be greater with bi-atrial MAZE procedures compared to PVI alone during CABG and or AVR [41, 42]. As with mitral surgery, performing the MAZE procedure during AVR and/or CABG surgery is also established to be safe [43]. SR restoration rates greater than 95% at 5 years have been reported following MAZE procedure and CABG, and concomitant PVI with CABG improves restoration of SR in paroxysmal AF, with SR rates greater than 85% at 18 months [41, 44]. The efficacy of surgical ablation following AVR and or CABG has been shown to be at least equivalent to, if not superior to that following mitral surgery [35, 45].

The European guidelines also advocate concomitant AF ablation during cardiac surgery and agree its safety [46, 47]. A variety of Class II recommendations are made [46]: (A) MAZE surgery, preferably bi-atrial, is recommended in symptomatic patients undergoing cardiac surgery to improve symptoms attributable to AF, balancing the added risk of the procedure and the benefit of rhythm control therapy. (B) Concomitant bi-atrial MAZE or PVI may be considered in asymptomatic AF patients undergoing cardiac surgery [48].

In stand-alone surgery, MAZE procedure via mini-thoracotomy or thoracoscopic PVI have shown success rates ranging from 60 to 85% at 1 year, and success following failed catheter ablation [49, 50]. European guidelines are positive, expressing that isolated epicardial PVI via minimally invasive surgery, OR MAZE surgery potentially using a minimally invasive approach should be considered, in patients with symptomatic refractory AF and failed catheter ablation.

Thoracoscopic ablation may be more effective in restoring SR than catheter ablation in selected patients, although rate of complications is higher in the surgically group [51, 52]. With ever improving ablation technology and surgical instrumentation, the ability to perform larger lesion sets via a minimally invasive approach is likely to increase; and lead to expansion in the use of stand-alone AF surgery, and hybrid surgical-electrophysiological ablation. Data relating to hybrid procedures is encouraging, with success rates greater than 80% at 1 year [53, 54]. Long procedure times currently impede greater use, and more evidence is required to define optimal patient selection and long-term efficacy.

5.2 Limitations of evidence

The data discussed thus far is encouraging for surgical AF ablation. However, it is impossible to draw firm conclusions from the large amount of data relating to surgical AF ablation, with relation to survival, and definitive conclusions relating to efficacy, are hampered by the multi-level heterogeneity, with respect to lesion set performed, nature/duration of AF, patient population, follow up duration and definition/assessment of rhythm outcomes. Satisfactorily sized randomised trials, with standardised lesion sets, energy devices, uniform follow-up and rhythm assessment are needed to provide high level evidence; and are in progress.

A recent Cochrane review of 22 published trials concluded for patients with AF undergoing cardiac surgery, that concomitant AF surgery doubles the rate of freedom from AF/atrial arrhythmias while increasing the risk of permanent pacemaker (PPM) implantation. However, the authors described the available evidence as only moderate quality, and concluded that effects on mortality were uncertain. Significant heterogeneity was encountered amongst studies, but safety, stroke risk, and health-related quality of life were not affected by concomitant surgical AF ablation. No benefit of one type of AF ablation over another was demonstrated [47]. All included studies were rated as being at a high risk of bias in at least one assessed domain. The recently published AMAZE randomised trial from Papworth, re-established that surgical ablation increases the proportion of patients in SR at 12 months and 24 months: 61.5% versus 46.9% and 58.5% versus 36.4%, respectively. The trialists concluded that surgical ablation was safe, but it did not improve quality of life or survival at 2 years, a relatively early time point. There was no significant difference in stroke-free survival, in serious adverse events, operative or overall survival, cardioversion or PPM implantation [55]. A major limitation of this study is that lesion sets were *not* standardised between surgeons. The longer-term results are awaited.

5.3 Pulmonary vein isolation versus MAZE procedure

The majority of surgical ablation studies in stand-alone AF have employed minimally invasive approaches; most frequently thoracoscopic off-pump RF PVI plus LAA amputation. Overall rates of freedom from AF of approximately 70–85% are reported at 12 months. Most studies, but not all, show conversion rates to be higher in paroxysmal AF than persistent AF when using PVI [56–58]. It is generally accepted that PVI is a reasonable treatment for paroxysmal AF with freedom rates of 70% reported at 5 years [59]. Direct randomised comparison between PVI and MAZE procedures is hard to find, with studies displaying marked heterogeneity.

In non-paroxysmal AF, PVI alone does not seem to be sufficient for maintenance of SR. In permanent AF patients with LA dilatation and valvular disease, additional lesions seem necessary. Systematic review of multiple studies shows that isolated PVI, has inferior efficacy to on-pump endocardial MAZE procedures, in patients with stand-alone AF, with a clear advantage of performing additional atrial lesions [60]. These effects are echoed in non-stand-alone AF. In a recent study of 260 patients undergoing mitral valve surgery, with pre-dominantly non-paroxysmal AF, patients underwent surgical ablation with either PVI or biatrial MAZE, or mitral valve surgery alone. At, 12 months post-surgery, both ablation groups showed lower rates of AF than those undergoing mitral valve surgeries alone. A higher rate of AF was seen in the PVI group compared to biatrial MAZE (36% versus 23%). The aim of this study was primarily to assess a novel rhythm monitoring strategy post-surgery, and not lesion set comparison. The trial was not powered to detect a difference between the PVI and biatrial MAZE, but re-enforced other studies findings that a more complete lesion set may be superior in restoring SR, in patients undergoing mitral valve surgery [61]. In patients undergoing aortic or mitral valve surgery with permanent AF, PVI alone has been shown to be significantly inferior to PVI + additional LA lesions in restoration of SR; 25% versus 86% at 2 years [62]. This study along with others has demonstrated via electrophysiological mapping that complete continuous isolation of the pulmonary veins is often not achieved during surgical ablation. In a combined population of paroxysmal and persistent AF patients undergoing the Cox-Maze IV procedure, superior freedom from AF was obtained when patients received complete posterior LA isolation via a box-lesion, compared to a line between the inferior PVs only. Patients received a variety of concomitant procedures in this study including; CABG, mitral valve repair, tricuspid valve replacement, closure of patent foramen and aortic valve replacement [63]. Gillinov et al. showed in a randomised mitral valve surgical population with persistent or long-standing persistent AF that surgical ablation significantly improved freedom from AF at 1 year [64]. In a sub-set analysis they showed that PVI alone in comparison to biatrial lesion set creation appeared to show equivalent results; approximately 60% freedom from AF at 1 year. The authors have commented that the study was not adequately powered to show a difference between the two ablation sets, and emphasised the need for larger randomised studies to explore this question. This study has also received criticism for the relatively low percentage use of bipolar RFA in the PVI group (43%), relatively low success rate of freedom from AF at 1 year (60%), and the creation of biatrial lesion sets that did not strictly adhere to the true MAZE concept. The latter criticism, coupled to the factor that adequacy of PVI was confirmed electrophyisologically intra-operatively, may have led to the enhanced efficacy of PVI seen in this study, in this population.

5.4 Post-operative and peri-operative drug therapy

5.4.1 Anticoagulation

Following surgical AF ablation, full anticoagulation is common and reasonable until durable restoration of SR is proven, as long as safety criteria for anticoagulation are met. Anticoagulation is usually continued until stable SR is documented by the very least 24-h Holter monitoring. The time point at which monitoring should be conducted is debated, but is commonly at the 6 month follow up point, but many advocate rhythm monitoring at 1 year or beyond, and at multiple time points to capture late recurrence [35]. Sensible practice also recommends an echocardiogram before discontinuing anticoagulation to confirm adequate LA emptying.

5.4.2 Anti-arrhythmic therapy

There are currently no guideline recommendations for specific anti-arrhythmic drug therapy following surgical ablation. Randomised, controlled, prospective data relating to this question is lacking and is desirable. As discussed earlier there is marked heterogeneity between surgical ablation studies, and this extends to definition of AF recurrence, rhythm assessment protocols and also anti-arrhythmic therapy. Forming firm conclusions based on these studies relating to optimal drug therapy regimens, would be non-scientific and inappropriate. For example, in the recently performed AMAZE trial, amiodarone use in the post-operative period was standardised; however, beta blocker use was left up to the discretion of treating teams [55].

Overall, anti-arrhythmic drug therapy is commonly given for 8–12 weeks after catheter or surgical ablation to reduce early AF recurrence. In addition, a 3 month immediate 'blanking period', in which rhythm assessment is not performed, is usually employed. A recent controlled trial in a catheter ablation population showed that amiodarone halved early AF recurrences compared with placebo [65].

The ESC guidelines on the management of AF raise the concern that prospective studies are lacking with relation to anti-arrhythmic therapy post-catheter ablation, and available evidence is weak [46]. They conclude that better AF prevention is afforded after catheter ablation with anti-arrhythmic therapy, and this represents reasonable practice. Review of the literature relating to surgical ablation reveals that this sensible practice is employed almost universally. AF conversion is generally measured by the percent of patients off class I or III antiarrhythmic drugs and free of atrial tachyarrhythmia at 3, 6, 9, 12, and 24 months postoperatively. Recurrence is generally defined as any atrial tachyarrhythmia lasting longer than 30 s on a 24-h Holter monitor recording 6 months after surgical ablation. Amiodarone is the most commonly used drug for enhancing rhythm control post-surgical ablation, although routine use is not universal. Concomitant use of beta-blockade is common, although, not always routine. A multitude of data exists relating to the likely benefits of statins, amiodarone and various other drug regimens in the prevention of post-operative AF during routine cardiac surgery. To extrapolate this data to the surgical AF ablation population is reasonable. However, detailed, controlled studies are needed to define the precise short and long-term impact of drug therapy following surgical ablation procedures. Specific delineation of differences between different populations, e.g. CABG versus valvular disease groups, and differing drug regimens is necessary, but maybe challenging. The lack of definite evidence relating to drug therapy is reflected by the STS recommendation for multidisciplinary heart team assessment and long-term follow up to optimise outcomes of surgical ablation for AF [35].

5.5 Animal studies

Safety and feasibility of surgical ablation technology and techniques was first explored in animal studies. The animal studies described here, stem from the efforts made to firstly (A) transition away from the traditional, technically demanding cut and sew MAZE procedure, as well as to (B) develop quicker, less invasive, +/– beating heart, surgical ablation techniques.

The limitations of animal studies with relation to extrapolation of efficacy to humans must be borne in mind. There are known differences in atrial tissue and epicardial fat thickness, between the various used animal species and humans. Atrial thickness in the domestic pig is similar to that of the human, but levels of epicardial fat in the human are significantly greater, and so too is the thickness of diseased human atria [66]. In addition, electrophysiological differences with relation to impulse generation and AF pathophysiology, varies between animal species and humans. As with human studies, a multitude of devices and lesion sets have been employed, utilising both normal and chronically fibrillating hearts, precluding direct meaningful study comparison. As such, specific animal studies clearly demonstrating efficacy of the MAZE procedure in restoration of SR are lacking. Overall, animal studies are best regarded as the preliminary studies that proved concept, safety and feasibility of surgical ablation in humans. They crucially provided the anatomical basis, technological characteristics/limitations, mechanistic insights and electrophysiological knowledge, which allowed informed ablation use in humans.

An early sheep study clearly established RFA to produce equally effective lesions to the cut and sew surgical technique. The RFA technique was shown to be significantly faster than incision technique with equivalent safety. In this 18 sheep, on-CPB endocardial ablation study, adequate lesion transmurality was demonstrated using pacing at both acute and chronic (1 month) time points. The lesion set performed was similar but not identical to the classical MAZE procedure, and this study amongst others established RFA to be a simple, time saving alternative to surgical incisions during open heart MAZE procedures [67].

Examination of a variety of ablation technology devices, in various porcine beating heart ablation models, highlighted large variation in their ability to achieve transmurality [66]. The majority of devices failed to achieve full thickness lesions, a factor along with lesion continuity that has proven critical in preventing AF recurrence. Overall, the most consistently reliable devices for creating transmural lesions were demonstrated to be bipolar RFA clamps [68]. Although, highly reliable when performing PVI, use in creating intra-cardiac lesions during beating heart surgery is restricted to the right side, due to potential catastrophic effects of air embolism on the left. As such, the majority of beating heart animal studies study epicardial devices. Porcine studies amongst others, helped delineate the challenges facing surgical epicardial ablation. These included variability of atrial wall muscle thickness and epicardial fat distribution, enhanced heat insulation by fat, and circulating intra-cavitary blood action as a potential heat sink [66]. These studies also identified the anatomical variation in reliability of transmurality achievement. Zones of difficulty, over Bachmann's bundle, crista terminalis and at the mitral or tricuspid annuli, LAA and RAA were identified, along with zones of higher success around the pulmonary veins [69].

Acute and chronic studies using bipolar RF epicardial lesions have established that they do not significantly change pulmonary vein flow, nor cause significant acute or chronic pulmonary vein stenosis [68, 70]. In addition, pacing and epicardial mapping have both confirmed consistent, successful bidirectional isolation, with the real-time tissue conductance assessment, being able to reliably predict short and long term transmurality. Histologic examination re-enforced safety, showing safe discrete lesions without evidence of stricture, or aneurysm formation [70].

6. Complications of atrial fibrillation surgery

A disputed aspect surrounding surgical AF ablation is that of the relationship to PPM insertion. The rate of PPM insertion following surgical AF ablation varies between 6% and 19%. The relationship is unclear, large meta-analyses comparing PPM insertion rates have demonstrated no significant increase in post-operative PPM requirement during concomitant AF ablation [48], yet a Cochrane review has demonstrated an increased requirement [47]. There is a presumed association between RA lesions and PPM implantation, and indeed a recent meta-analysis demonstrated that bi-atrial AF ablation surgery was associated with increased PPM insertion compared to isolated LA ablation [71]. Although not universal, most clinical studies show the increased need for PPM after AF ablation surgery to be driven mainly by sick sinus syndrome [9]. A proposed possible explanation is that of unmasking preoperative sinus node dysfunction. However, due to a multitude of confounding variables and lack of accurate reporting of preoperative data, it is not possible to precisely establish a causal mechanism.

As discussed earlier, despite increased CPB time and hospital length of stay, in the modern era, concomitant surgical AF ablation is regarded as safe, with no increase in mortality demonstrated [47, 72]. In addition, most studies demonstrate no increase in peri-operative stroke [47, 72]. Overall, the frequency of cardiac tamponade, pericardial effusion, myocardial infarction and re-operative bleeding does not appear to increase following concomitant surgical AF ablation [47, 72]. With relation to minimally invasive MAZE procedures and surgical AF ablation for stand-alone AF, safety is also acceptable. Minimally invasive epicardial surgical ablation is perceived to be safer than the endocardial MAZE procedure, because the former requires smaller incisions and does not require CPB. However, no statistically significant difference in mortality has been demonstrated [73]. Mortality rates of less than 0.5% are reported [60]. Results vary and are technique dependent, with some analyses showing lower re-operative bleeding rates and conversion to sternotomy with minimally invasive endocardial MAZE procedure [60], and others favouring minimally invasive epicardial surgical ablation without the use of CPB [73]. Similar conflicting results are noted with respect to the incidence of renal failure and hospital length of stay. As mentioned earlier, controlled studies are required to precisely delineate relationships between efficacy and safety of various minimally invasive techniques.

6.1 Predictors of AF recurrence following surgical ablation

Great efforts have been directed towards identifying predictors of AF recurrence, but have been hampered by the heterogeneity of studies with relation to ablation set, AF characteristics, rhythm assessment and pharmacological regimens, amongst other variables. Risk factors for recurrence are broadly classified into pre-operative variables and intra-operative variables. Preoperative variables associated with AF recurrence include increasing LA diameter [15, 74, 75], age [76], and prolonged pre-operative duration of AF [75, 76]. In an excellent 280 patient prospective study, Damiano et al. showed in patients with both paroxysmal AF and persistent AF three risk factors for AF recurrence following the MAZE IV procedure: increasing LA size, early post-operative AF and failure to anatomically isolate the entire posterior LA [15]. LA size of over 8 cm being has been shown by the same group to correlate with a >50% chance of AF recurrence. Gillinov et al. also showed in approximately 260 patients undergoing the cut and sew MAZE III procedure and mitral valve surgery, in a cohort of predominantly permanent AF patients, that risk factors for AF recurrence included longer duration of AF, larger LA diameter, older age, and higher left ventricular mass index [76]. *In a systematic review involving 5200 patients from 19 studies the authors showed that AF recurrence after surgical ablation was again most often predicted by LA size, duration of AF and age* [75]. *They also concluded that the* innate heterogeneity of published data precluded a meta-analysis for predictors of surgical ablation success, and highlighted the need for consistent and reliable outcome predictors, and a standardised system of measurement for clinical parameters.

Impact of intra-operative variables such as energy source and lesion set are a contested area. Again, heterogeneity of studies hinders comparison. Overall it is difficult to demonstrate that use of various energy sources affects AF recurrence rates. Similar long-term success rates have been observed with either uni- or bipolar RFA and cryoablation [77], yet both superiority of either bipolar RFA [78] or monopolar [79] has been shown in different studies. Although not certain, the bi-atrial lesion set appears to display superiority to isolated LA lesion set in prevention of AF recurrence [78, 80]. In addition, modifiable risk factors such as hypertension, diabetes and smoking are implicated in surgical ablation failure [81].

7. Surgical versus catheter ablation

Catheter ablation is highly effective for the treatment of symptomatic, drug refractory AF. The reported efficacy for catheter ablation varies widely, although freedom from AF of up to 70% is reported, with worldwide registry data showing a procedural major adverse event rate of ~ 4.5%. Catheter ablation for the treatment of AF is currently recommended by guidelines as a second-line therapy in patients with paroxysmal and persistent AF after treatment with ≥1 antiarrhythmic drug has failed (Class I recommendation for paroxysmal AF, Class IIa for persistent AF, and Class IIb for long-stranding persistent). Most randomised controlled trials (RCTs) of drug therapy versus catheter ablation have studied patients with preserved left ventricular function [82]. Recently, RCTs have also shown the benefit of rhythm control with catheter ablation over medical therapy for AF associated with heart failure [83]. A recent meta-analysis examining six RCTs confirmed these findings demonstrating catheter ablation to be superior to medical therapy for AF in patients with HF, resulting in greater improvement in LVEF, quality of life and functional status, with a definite survival benefit [84]. Results from the recent CABANA trial also echo these positive catheter ablation effects in HF patients [85]. Although variable, a pooled freedom from AF of 71% was seen in this analysis.

There is not much direct comparison of surgical ablation versus catheter ablation in the literature. The FAST study included 124 patients with drug–refractory AF, LA dilatation and hypertension or failed prior catheter ablation. Patients were randomised to either catheter ablation or thoracoscopic surgical ablation. Catheter ablation consisted of linear antral PVI and optional additional lines. Surgical ablation consisted of bipolar RF PVI, ganglionated plexi ablation, and LAA excision with optional additional lines. Freedom from AF was superior for surgical ablation at 12 months (36.5% versus 65.6%), but this was at the expense of greater rate of complications, driven mainly by pneumothorax, major bleeding, and the need for PPM [52]. A meta-analysis of eight studies showed that thoracoscopic surgical ablation showed significantly greater freedom from AF at 12-months compared to catheter ablation (78.4 versus 53%), with a reduced requirement for repeat ablation [86]. This superiority was maintained in paroxysmal and persistent AF subgroups. However, again, complications were shown to be considerably higher in the surgical group, driven mainly by pleural effusion and pneumothorax. Limitations of the data were the retrospective nature of some of the included studies and the heterogeneity of patients involved.

The superior efficacy demonstrated by surgical intervention is postulated to be due to several factors [86]. The ablation lesion set employed with surgery is generally much more extensive including PVI, but also targeted epicardial ganglionic plexi, LAA excision and additional LA lines. The importance of ganglionic plexi and the LAA in perpetuating AF re-entrant circuits is well recognised [87, 88]. In catheter ablation relative inadequate treatment may be occurring, as additional ablation lines are often not performed, with endocardial lesions consisting of PVI using wide-area antrum ablation alone. In addition, a better ability of surgical technology to create adequate transmural lesions may underlie its superior efficacy.

Debate continues regarding the optimal lesion set for stand-alone surgical ablation. Specifically, the comparative efficacy of strategies of PVI versus extended LA lesion sets, or MAZE IV approach remains unknown, and requires further study. Further controlled studies are also needed to delineate the apparent supremacy of surgical ablation over catheter ablation. However, concerns relating to the higher rate of complications and prolonged length of stay of the more invasive surgical approach currently impede adoption of its use on a broader scale. The majority of these complications are non-severe and managed conservatively, and whether such this level of apprehension is justified is unclear. Surgical ablation is increasingly performed as a stand-alone procedure and with improving technology and surgical skill its use is likely to expand with time, either on its own or as part of a hybrid electrophysiological approach.

7.1 Electrophysiological mapping

Unfortunately electrophysiological evaluation after bipolar RF PV isolation has been scarcely performed. Only a small minority of surgical ablation studies have performed detailed intra-operative or peri-operative validation of ablation sets [64]. It is clear that confirmation of adequacy of ablation transmurality and continuity impacts upon surgical ablation efficacy and subsequent AF recurrence rate [89, 90]. Several factors oppose routine electrophysiological validation of ablation including; (A) technically challenging to adequately pace in between instead of on the performed ablation lines, (B) time consuming to perform correctly; with epicardial lesions, at least 20 min between PV isolation and endocardial validation is needed and (C) precise delineation of the border between conducting and non-conducting tissue at the distal sleeve of the PV is sometimes difficult to perform without complex mapping techniques. In its simplest form following PVI, entrance block is defined as failure to capture the PVs during pacing from the LA, and exit block can be defined by failure to capture the LA, when pacing from the PVs distal to the RF lesions.

Following minimally invasive PVI, recurrence rates as high as 40% have been seen despite intra-operative electrophysiological validation. Repeat electrophysiological investigation shows the vast majority are due to PV reconnection. In mini-MAZE [90] and total thoracoscopic procedures [91] intra-operative electrophysiological validation has been associated with higher success rates of 84% and 93% at 24 and 12 months respectively, in mixed AF populations. Sophisticated 3D electrophysiological mapping again showed recurrence was secondary to PV gaps in 50% of patients, with ectopic foci in LAA, peri-mitral LA roof flutter in the remainder. Post-operative recurrence is generally amenable to catheter ablation, with good intermediate-term success [92]. These findings re-enforce the growing belief that the hybrid ablation approach, either immediate or staged will produce the best long term ablation outcomes. Augmented success rates with a combined staged hybrid approach have been achieved, with a required catheter-based 'touch up' rate of approximately 20% following surgical intervention [93].

The predominant factor in AF recurrence post-ablation is PV reconnection or incomplete isolation. Several reasons for the gaps around the PVI ring are implicated: (A) clamp application failure over the roof of the superior PVs, (B) incomplete clamping at the bottom of inferior PV, (C) clamp application failure at the antral side of the PV due to the long distance between the superior and inferior PVs, or accessory PVs and (D) increasing LA size. Multiple reasons for improper clamp application and diminished RFA effect are also cited including (A) angulation of clamps rather than perpendicular placement; (B) blood within the PVs limiting tissue involution between the clamps on beating hearts; (C) clamp movement during beating heart ablation; (D) the cooling effect of circulating blood and (E) anatomic factors such as atrial folds, ridges and variable myocardial thickness.

Improving the quality of the lesion set, will undoubtedly improve durability and success of surgical ablation; and better intra-operative electrophysiological mapping strategies represents a good target to focus upon. It is clear that simple entrance and exit block confirmation has a false negative rate, most likely related to tissue oedema, trauma and ischaemia, and the optimum universal mapping technique and strategy is not established. Randomised controlled studies with detailed electrophysiological interrogation follow up, are needed to identify this technique and strategy and then standardise their application, and improve surgical lesion set creation.

8. Left atrial appendage intervention

LAA exclusion or occlusion LAAO can be safely performed. Growing interest in LAA intervention has been driven by the observation that 90% of thrombi in non-valvular AF (NVAF) and 60% of those in valvular AF develop in the LAA. LAAO by surgical excision or device occlusion is postulated to reduce the risk of stroke, peripheral thromboemboli, and necessity for oral anticoagulants. Surgical techniques available to isolate the LAA include LAA excision with amputation, or occlusion which can be performed endocardially or epicardially. LAAO can be performed using an implantable device or without. Non-device approaches include surgical two-layer closure with running or mattress sutures, stapling and excision, and placement of surgical purse-strings or clips around the LAA base. Success is dependent on total LAA excision or isolation. Any residual stump of the LAA >1 cm in length, or gap with associated blood flow is thrombogenic [94]. LAA exclusion however has been inconsistent in terms of techniques, rates of complete exclusion, and thus adoption. Studies comparing internal ligation, external staple excision and surgical excision show that complete LAA elimination should not be assumed. Initial stump-free elimination can deteriorate with time, and a residual stump can be immediately present, emphasising the importance of immediate and late echocardiographic interrogation of LAA intervention [95].

8.1 Left atrial appendage devices

A variety of devices exist. The most widely used endocardial device is the Watchman device, which is a percutaneously delivered polyester fabric on a nitinol frame (**Figure 10**). The Lariat device utilises a combined percutaneous and epicardial approach to deliver a lasso around the appendage guided by an intraluminal magnet tip. The AtriClip is made of two polyester-covered parallel tubes with nitinol springs (**Figure 11**). The AtriClip is a self-closing clamp placed epicardially at the base of the LAA to exclude blood flow. In general, endocardial devices remain in contact with intracardiac blood, and therefore anticoagulation for 2 months is recommended following implantation, making them less attractive for patients with contraindications to anticoagulation. Endocardial devices also fail to lie properly in LAAs with unfavourable morphologies.

The strongest evidence supporting reduction of stroke risk and potentially the elimination of anticoagulation with LAAO comes from the large, multi-centre RCT, PROTECT AF. This study used the percutaneous Watchman LAA device. After

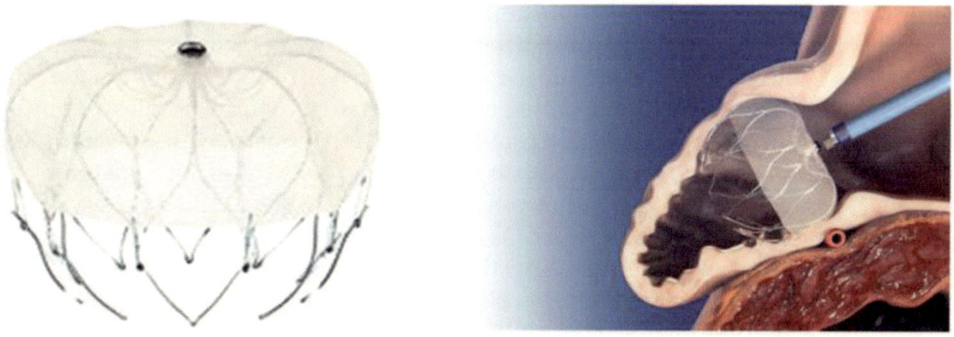

Figure 10.
The watchman left atrial appendage occlusion device. A percutaneously delivered polyester fabric device on a nitinol frame [108].

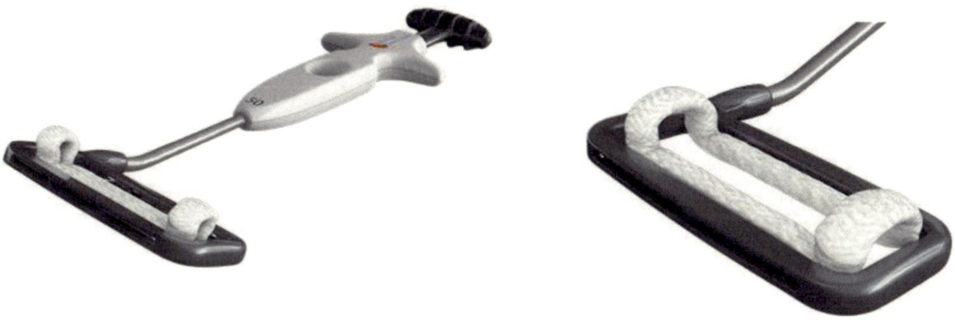

Figure 11.
Left atrial appendage occlusion AtriClip device. Parallel titanium crossbars apply adequate pressure without crushing or damaging tissue [105].

3.8 years of follow-up in patients with NVAF at elevated risk for stroke, percutaneous LAA closure met criteria for both non-inferiority and superiority, compared with warfarin, for preventing the combined outcome of stroke, systemic embolism, and cardiovascular death, as well as superiority for cardiovascular and all-cause mortality [96].

In a large meta-analysis reviewing over 2400 patients, the efficacy of LAA closure compared to warfarin in 2 RCTS, PREVENT AF and the PREVAIL trial was analysed. At a mean follow up of 2.7 years in patients with NVAF at increased risk for stroke or bleeding, LAA intervention improved rates of haemorrhagic stroke, cardiovascular/unexplained death, and non-procedural bleeding. These positive effects were offset by an increase in ischemic strokes, mainly peri-procedural. All-cause stroke or systemic embolism was similar between both strategies. This analysis emphasised a non-inferiority of LAAO to warfarin use; with LAA intervention beneficial effects seeming to be underpinned by the circumvention of anticoagulation-related morbidity and mortality, as opposed to prevention of thromboembolism [97]. However, these positive results could not be automatically extrapolated to surgical LAA intervention.

8.2 Left atrial appendage intervention during cardiac surgery

Retrospective analysis of over 10,000 patients undergoing surgical AF ablation with and without concomitant surgical LAAO, showed only 37% underwent LAAO. Concomitant LAAO significantly reduced readmission for thromboembolism and all-cause mortality. The additional procedure was demonstrated to be safe, but the important differentiation between technique of LAAO, nature of AF and echocardiographic parameters between groups was not made [98]. In an updated meta-analysis examining over 3600 patients from 7 studies a significant reduction in stroke, and all-cause mortality was demonstrated in patients with AF undergoing LAAO during cardiac surgery, compared to those not undergoing LAAO. Techniques of suture ligation and stapling were utilised, and a variety of post-operative anticoagulation regimens and follow up periods [99].

The best clinical evidence for LAAO devices exists for the AtriClip device (AtriCure). It is the most commonly used surgical device with over 100,000 recorded implants worldwide. It is applied with concomitant cardiac operations as well as in isolated thoracoscopic procedures safety and efficacy of the AtriClip device was evaluated in the EXCLUDE trial. In 70 patients undergoing primary cardiac operations AtriClip, demonstrated 95% successful exclusion with 98% complete LAA exclusion on CT at 3 months [100]. Success was defined as occlusion with no residual neck >1 cm and no leaks or migration. The upcoming results of the large (n = 4700) multicentre, randomised LAAOS III trial will aid in clarifying the long-term outcomes of LAAO in AF patients undergoing cardiac surgery [101].

The practice of prophylactic LAA closure in patients without AF undergoing cardiac surgery does not appear to be effective. A recent large scale, propensity-matched analysis of prophylactic LAA closure, showed that this was associated with early increase in post-operative AF and no decrease in stroke risk or mortality [102]. The ATLAS trial is now randomising patients without documented AF, at high risk for the developing post-operative AF undergoing elective cardiac surgery; to LAA exclusion with the AtriClip or no concomitant AtriClip placement. The LAAOS III and ATLAS trials are the largest trials investigating efficacy of LAA occlusion for stroke prevention at the time of cardiac surgery; and their results are eagerly awaited.

Currently, the US and the European guidelines state that it is reasonable to, or consideration should be given to, performing LAA intervention in conjunction with surgical AF ablation and during cardiac surgery, for longitudinal thromboembolic morbidity prevention (Class II, Level C/B). European guidelines also say it is reasonable to perform isolated LAA intervention in patients in AF with contraindication to anticoagulation.

8.3 Left atrial appendage intervention and anticoagulation

There is large variability in anticoagulation strategies post LAAO and surgical ablation alone with mixed-use of warfarin, NOACs and single and dual antiplatelet agents. The optimal anticoagulation therapy is still a matter of debate. Decisions regarding anticoagulation and imaging should be made and tailored to patient and procedural characteristics. The decision is often straight forward, in patients with a contraindication to anticoagulation referred for LAA exclusion. However, for patients without contraindications to anticoagulation, the decision is less simple. The Zurich group has shown in 36 patients receiving AtriClip, with a mean CHA2DS2-VASc score of 3.7, that only one transient ischemic attack (TIA) occurred after >1200 day follow up, with no strokes [98]. Three patients received anticoagulation. They have also shown a reduction in stroke risk in 291 patients with a mean CHA2DS2-VASc score of 3.1, receiving AtriClip during concomitant surgery cardiac surgery [103]. Patients that did not receive anticoagulation after LAA exclusion had a relative risk reduction of 87.5% in stroke, with an observed ischaemic stroke-rate of 0.5/100 patient-years compared with an expected rate in a group of patients with similar CHA2DS2-VASc scores of 4.0/100 patient-years. No evidence of reperfusion or residual stump was observed [104].

Evidence regarding anticoagulation management post-operatively is not robust, and further well-powered long-term evidence is needed to confidently guide anticoagulation management in patients receiving the AtriClip but have no contraindications to anticoagulation. Currently, the European guidelines recommend that patients undergoing LAA intervention remain on anticoagulation (Class 1). However, the view that anticoagulation is not needed after AtriClip application is also held by many, with single anti-platelet agent thought to be sufficient.

9. Summary and conclusions

Surgical AF ablation has evolved over the past few decades and is now safe, and associated with minimal morbidity. The gold standard lesion set remains that of the MAZE IV, yet 'lesser' lesion sets, are gaining favour within the minimally invasive, hybrid and non-hybrid treatment setting, for treatment of NVAF. It is clear that surgical ablation displays beneficial effects, but the supportive evidence is not of the highest quality, and high quality RCTS with standardised ablation sets, AF criteria and defined rhythm assessment outcomes are needed. New studies need to precisely define and quantify the role of surgical ablation on rhythm, survival, symptoms, thromboembolic risk, and the exact relationship with specific target AF populations. Similarly, high level evidence is needed to quantify the impact of LAA intervention on thromboembolic risk in AF. Identification of the optimal LAA intervention, together with clear guidance on anticoagulation is necessary.

Author details

Manoraj Navaratnarajah*, Suvitesh Luthra and Sunil Ohri
Department of Cardiac Surgery, University Hospital Southampton, Southampton, Hampshire, United Kingdom

*Address all correspondence to: manoraj.navaratnarajah@doctors.org.uk

References

[1] Xu J, Luc JG, Phan K. Atrial fibrillation: Review of current treatment strategies. Journal of Thoracic Disease. 2016;**8**(9):E886-E900

[2] Menezes AR, Lavie CJ, DiNicolantonio JJ, et al. Atrial fibrillation in the 21st century: A current understanding of risk factors and primary prevention strategies. Mayo Clinic Proceedings. 2013;**88**:394-409

[3] Svennberg E, Engdahl J, Al-Khalili F, et al. Mass screening for untreated atrial fibrillation: The STROKESTOP study. Circulation. 2015;**131**:2176-2184

[4] Heeringa J, van der Kuip DA, Hofman A, et al. Prevalence, incidence and lifetime risk of atrial fibrillation: The Rotterdam study. European Heart Journal. 2006;**27**:949-953

[5] Eguchi K, Ohtaki E, Matsumura T, et al. Pre-operative atrial fibrillation as the key determinant of outcome of mitral valve repair for degenerative mitral regurgitation. European Heart Journal. 2005;**26**:1866-1872

[6] Lim E, Barlow CW, Hosseinpour AR, et al. Influence of atrial fibrillation on outcome following mitral valve repair. Circulation. 2001;**104**:I59-I63

[7] Maan A, Heist EK, Passeri J, et al. Impact of atrial fibrillation on outcomes in patients who underwent transcatheter aortic valve replacement. The American Journal of Cardiology. 2015;**115**:220-226

[8] Geidel S, Lass M, Boczor S, et al. Monopolar and bipolar radiofrequency ablation surgery: 3-Year experience in 90 patients with permanent atrial fibrillation. The Heart Surgery Forum. 2004;7:E398-E402

[9] Gammie JS, Haddad M, Milford-Beland S, et al. Atrial fibrillation correction surgery: Lessons from the Society of Thoracic Surgeons National Cardiac Database. The Annals of Thoracic Surgery. 2008;**85**:909-914

[10] Ad N, Suri RM, Gammie JS, et al. Surgical ablation of atrial fibrillation trends and outcomes in North America. The Journal of Thoracic and Cardiovascular Surgery. 2012;**144**:1051-1060

[11] Cox JL. Atrial fibrillation II: Rationale for surgical treatment. The Journal of Thoracic and Cardiovascular Surgery. 2003;**126**(6):1693-1699

[12] Cox JL. The surgical management of cardiac arrhythmias. Cardiovascular Clinics. 1987;**17**:381-413

[13] Cox JL, Churyla A, Malaisrie SC, Kruse J, et al. When is a MAZE procedure a MAZE procedure? The Canadian Journal of Cardiology. 2018;**34**(11):1482-1491

[14] Cox JL, Jaquiss RD, Schuessler RB, et al. Modification of the Maze procedure for atrial flutter and atrial fibrillation: II. Surgical technique of the Maze III procedure. Journal of Thoracic and Cardiovascular Surger. 1995;**110**(2):485-495

[15] Damiano RJ Jr, Schwartz FH, Bailey MS, et al. The Cox Maze IV procedure: Predictors of late recurrence. The Journal of Thoracic and Cardiovascular Surgery. 2011;**141**:113-121

[16] Johansson B, Houltz B, Berglin E, et al. Shortterm sinus rhythm predicts longterm sinus rhythm and clinical improvement after intraoperative ablation of atrial fibrillation. Europace. 2008;**10**:610-617

[17] Khargi K, Lemke B, Deneke T. Concomitant antiarrhythmic procedures to treat permanent atrial fibrillation in

CABG and AVR patients are as effective as in mitral valve patients. European Journal of Cardio-Thoracic Surgery. 2005;**27**:841-846

[18] Beukema WP, Sie HT, Misier AR, et al. Intermediate to longterm results of radiofrequency modified Maze procedure as an adjunct to openheart surgery. The Annals of Thoracic Surgery. 2008;**86**:1409-1414

[19] Chiappini B, Di Bartolomeo R, Marinelli G. Radiofrequency ablation for atrial fibrillation: Different approaches. Asian Cardiovascular & Thoracic Annals. 2004;**12**:272-277

[20] von Oppell UO, Masani N, O'Callaghan P, et al. Mitral valve surgery plus concomitant atrial fibrillation ablation is superior to mitral valve surgery alone with an intensive rhythm control strategy. European Journal of Cardio-Thoracic Surgery. 2009;**35**:641-650

[21] Basu S, Nagendran M, Maruthappu M. How effective is bipolar radiofrequency ablation for atrial fibrillation during concomitant cardiac surgery? Interactive Cardiovascular and Thoracic Surgery. 2012;**15**:741-748

[22] Camm CF, Nagendran M, Xiu PY, et al. How effective is cryoablation for atrial fibrillation during concomitant cardiac surgery? Interactive Cardiovascular and Thoracic Surgery. 2011;**13**:410-414

[23] Blomström-Lundqvist C, Johansson B, Berglin E, et al. A randomized doubleblind study of epicardial left atrial cryoablation for permanent atrial fibrillation in patients undergoing mitral valve surgery: The SWEDish Multicentre Atrial Fibrillation Study (SWEDMAF). European Heart Journal. 2007;**28**:2902-2908

[24] MacDonald DR, Maruthappu M, Nagendran M. How effective is microwave ablation for atrial fibrillation during concomitant cardiac surgery? Interactive Cardiovascular and Thoracic Surgery. 2012;**15**:122-127

[25] Lin Z, Shan ZG, Liao CX, et al. The effect of microwave and bipolar radiofrequency ablation in the surgical treatment of permanent atrial fibrillation during valve surgery. The Thoracic and Cardiovascular Surgeon. 2011;**59**:460-464

[26] Kim JB, Cho WC, Jung SH, et al. Alternative energy sources for surgical treatment of atrial fibrillation in patients undergoing mitral valve surgery: Microwave ablation vs cryoablation. Journal of Korean Medical Science. 2010;**25**:1467-1472

[27] Kyprianou K, Pericleous A, Stavrou A, et al. Surgical perspectives in the management of atrial fibrillation. World Journal of Cardiology. 2016;**8**(1):41-56

[28] Klinkenberg TJ, Ahmed S, Ten Hagen A, et al. Feasibility and outcome of epicardial pulmonary vein isolation for lone atrial fibrillation using minimal invasive surgery and high intensity focused ultrasound. Europace. 2009;**11**:1624-1631

[29] Schmidt B, Chun KR, Metzner A, et al. Pulmonary vein isolation with highintensity focused ultrasound: Results from the HIFU 12F study. Europace. 2009;**11**:1281-1288

[30] Lawrance CP, Henn MC, Damiano RJ Jr. Surgical ablation for atrial fibrillation: Techniques, indications, and results. Current Opinion in Cardiology. 2015 Jan;**30**(1):58-64

[31] van Laar C, Kelder J, van Putte BP. The totally thoracoscopic maze procedure for the treatment of atrial fibrillation. Interactive Cardiovascular and Thoracic Surgery. 2017 Jan;**24**(1):102-111

[32] Yilmaz A, Geuzebroek GS, Van Putte BP, et al. Completely

thoracoscopic pulmonary vein isolation with ganglionic plexus ablation and left atrial appendage amputation for treatment of atrial fibrillation. European Journal of Cardio-Thoracic Surgery. 2010;**38**(3):356-360

[33] Vos LM, Bentala M, Geuzebroek GS, et al. Long-term outcome after totally thoracoscopic ablation for atrial fibrillation. Journal of Cardiovascular Electrophysiology. Jan 2020;**31**(1):40-45

[34] Osmancik P, Budera P, Zdarska J, et al. Electrophysiological findings after surgical thoracoscopic atrial fibrillation ablation. Heart Rhythm. 2016;**13**(6):1246-1252

[35] Badhwar V, Rankin JS, Damiano RJ Jr, et al. The Society of Thoracic Surgeons 2017 clinical practice guidelines for the surgical treatment of atrial fibrillation. The Annals of Thoracic Surgery. 2017;**103**(1):329-341

[36] Saint L, Damiano RJ, Cuculich PS, et al. Incremental risk of the Cox-maze IV procedure for patients with atrial fibrillation undergoing mitral valve surgery. The Journal of Thoracic and Cardiovascular Surgery. 2013;**146**:1072-1077

[37] Rankin JS, He X, O'Brien SM, et al. The Society of Thoracic Surgeons risk model for operative mortality after multiple valve surgery. The Annals of Thoracic Surgery. 2013;**95**:1484-1490

[38] Lee R, McCarthy PM, Wang EC, et al. Midterm survival inpatients treated for atrial fibrillation: A propensity-matched comparison to patients without a history of atrial fibrillation. The Journal of Thoracic and Cardiovascular Surgery. 2012;**143**:1341-1351

[39] Attaran S, Saleh HZ, Shaw M, et al. Does the outcome improve after radiofrequency ablation for atrial fibrillation in patients undergoing cardiac surgery? A propensity-matched comparison. European Journal of Cardio-Thoracic Surgery. 2012;**41**:806-811

[40] Saxena A, Dinh DT, Reid CM, et al. Does preoperative atrial fibrillation portend a poorer prognosis in patients undergoing isolated aortic valve replacement? A multicentre Australian study. The Canadian Journal of Cardiology. 2013;**29**:697-703

[41] Damiano RJ, Gaynor SL, Bailey M, et al. The long-term outcome of patients with coronary disease and atrial fibrillation undergoing the Cox maze procedure. The Journal of Thoracic and Cardiovascular Surgery. 2003;**126**:2016-2021

[42] Ad N, Henry L, Hunt S, et al. Do we increase the operative risk by adding the Cox maze III procedure to aortic valve replacement and coronary artery bypass surgery? The Journal of Thoracic and Cardiovascular Surgery. 2012;**143**:936-944

[43] Malaisrie SC, Lee R, Kruse J, et al. Atrial fibrillation ablation in patients undergoing aortic valve replacement. The Journal of Heart Valve Disease. 2012;**21**:350-357

[44] Pokushalov E, Romanov A, Corbucci G, et al. Benefit of ablation of first diagnosed paroxysmalatrial fibrillation during coronary artery bypass grafting: A pilot study. European Journal of Cardio-Thoracic Surgery. 2012;**41**:556-560

[45] Khargi K, Hutten BA, Lemke B, et al. Surgical treatment of atrial fibrillation; a systematic review. European Journal of Cardio-Thoracic Surgery. 2005;**27**:258-265

[46] Kirchhof P, Benussi S, Kotecha D, et al. ESC guidelines for the management of atrial fibrillation developed in collaboration with EACTS. European Heart Journal. 2016;**37**(38):2893-2962

[47] Huffman MD, Karmali KN, Berendsen MA, et al. Concomitant atrial fibrillation surgery for people undergoing cardiac surgery. Cochrane Database of Systematic Reviews. 2016;**8**:CD011814

[48] Cheng DC, Ad N, Martin J, et al. Surgical ablation for atrial fibrillation in cardiac surgery: A meta-analysis and systematic review. Innovations (Phila). 2010;**5**:84-96

[49] McClelland JH, Duke D, Reddy R. Preliminary results of a limited thoracotomy: New approach to treat atrial fibrillation. Journal of Cardiovascular Electrophysiology. 2007;**18**:1289-1295

[50] Castella M, Pereda D, Mestres CA, et al. Thoracoscopic pulmonary vein isolation in patients with atrial fibrillation and failed percutaneous ablation. The Journal of Thoracic and Cardiovascular Surgery. 2010;**140**:633-638

[51] Wang S, Liu L, Zou C. Comparative study of video-assisted thoracoscopic surgery ablation and radiofrequency catheter ablation on treating paroxysmal atrial fibrillation: A randomized, controlled short-term trial. Chinese Medical Journal. 2014;**127**:2567-2570

[52] Boersma LV, Castella M, van Boven W, et al. Atrial fibrillation catheter ablation versus surgical ablation treatment (FAST): A 2-center randomized clinical trial. Circulation. 2012;**125**:23-30

[53] Krul SP, Driessen AH, van Boven WJ, et al. Thoracoscopic video-assisted pulmonary vein antrum isolation, ganglionated plexus ablation, and periprocedural confirmation of ablation lesions: First results of a hybrid surgical electrophysiological approach for atrial fibrillation. Circulation. Arrhythmia and Electrophysiology. 2011;**4**:262-270

[54] La Meir M, Gelsomino S, Luca F, et al. Minimally invasive surgical treatment of lone atrial fibrillation: Early results of hybrid versus standard minimally invasive approach employing radiofrequency sources. International Journal of Cardiology. 2013;**167**:1469-1475

[55] Nashef SAM, Fynn S, Abu-Omar Y, et al. Amaze: A randomized controlled trial of adjunct surgery for atrial fibrillation. European Journal of Cardio-Thoracic Surgery. 1 Oct 2018;**54**(4):729-737

[56] Edgerton JR, McClelland JH, Duke D, et al. Minimally invasive surgical ablation of atrial fibrillation: Six-month results. The Journal of Thoracic and Cardiovascular Surgery. 2009;**138**:109-114

[57] Edgerton JR, Brinkman WT, Weaver T, et al. Pulmonary vein isolation and autonomic denervation for the management of paroxysmal atrial fibrillation by a minimally invasive surgical approach. The Journal of Thoracic and Cardiovascular Surgery. 2010;**140**:823-828

[58] Kasirajan V, Spradlin EA, Mormando TE, et al. Minimally invasive surgery using bipolar radiofrequency energy is effective treatment for refractory atrial fibrillation. The Annals of Thoracic Surgery. 2012;**93**:1456-1461

[59] De Maat Gijs E, Pozzoli A, et al. Long-term results of surgical minimally invasive pulmonary vein isolation for paroxysmal lone atrial fibrillation. Europace. 2015;**17**(5):747-752

[60] Je HG, Shuman DJ, Ad N. A systematic review of minimally invasive surgical treatment for atrial fibrillation: A comparison of the Cox-maze procedure, beating-heart epicardial ablation, and the hybrid procedure on safety and efficacy. European Journal of Cardio-Thoracic Surgery. 2015;**48**:531-541

[61] Blackstone EH, Chang HL, Rajeswaran J, et al. Biatrial maze procedure versus pulmonary vein isolation for atrial fibrillation during mitral valve surgery: New analytical approaches and end points. Journal of

Thoracic and Cardiovascular Surgery. 2019;**157**(1):234-243

[62] Gaita F, Riccardi R, Caponi D, et al. Linear cryoablation of the left atrium versus pulmonary vein cryoisolation in patients with permanent atrial fibrillation and valvular heart disease: Correlation of electroanatomic mapping and long-term clinical results. Circulation. 2005;**111**(2):136-142

[63] Voeller RK, Bailey MS, Zierer A, et al. Isolating the entire posterior left atrium improves surgical outcomes after the Cox maze procedure. The Journal of Thoracic and Cardiovascular Surgery. 2008;**135**(4):870-877

[64] Gillinov AM, Gelijns AC, Parides, et al. Surgical ablation of atrial fibrillation during mitral-valve surgery. The New England Journal of Medicine. 2015;**372**(15):1399-1409

[65] Darkner S, Chen X, Hansen J, et al. Recurrence of arrhythmia following short-term oral AMIOdarone after CATheter ablation for atrial fibrillation: A double-blind, randomized, placebo-controlled study (AMIO-CAT trial). European Heart Journal. 2014;**35**:3356-3364

[66] Schuessler RB, Lee AM, Melby SJ, et al. Animal studies of epicardial atrial ablation. Heart Rhythm. 2009;**6**(12 Suppl):S41-S45

[67] Caccitolo JA, Stulak JM, Schaff HV, et al. Open-heart endocardial radiofrequency ablation: An alternative to incisions in maze surgery. The Journal of Surgical Research. 2001;**97**(1):27-33

[68] Prasad SM, Maniar HS, Schuessler RB, et al. Chronic transmural atrial ablation by using bipolar radiofrequency energy on the beating heart. Journal of Thoracic & Cardiovascular Surgery. 2002;**124**(4):708-713

[69] Doll N, Kornherr P, Aupperle H, et al. Epicardial treatment of atrial fibrillation using cryoablation in an acute off-pump sheep model. The Thoracic and Cardiovascular Surgeon. 2003;**51**(5):267-273

[70] Prasad SM, Maniar HS, Diodata MD, et al. Physiological consequences of bipolar radiofrequency energy on the atria and pulmonary veins: A chronic animal study. Annals of Thoracic Surgery. 2003;**76**(3):836-841; discussion 841-2

[71] McClure GR, Belley-Cote EP, Jaffer IH, et al. Surgical ablation of atrial fibrillation: A systematic review and meta-analysis of randomized controlled trials. Europace. 2018;**20**(9):1442-1450

[72] Phan K, Xie A, Tian DH, Shaikhrezai K, Yan TD. Systematic review and meta-analysis of surgical ablation for atrial fibrillation during mitral valve surgery. Annals of Cardiothoracic Surgery. 2014;**3**(1):3-14

[73] Ad N, Suri RM, Gammie JS, Sheng S, O'Brien SM, Henry L. Surgical ablation of atrial fibrillation trends and outcomes in North America. The Journal of Thoracic and Cardiovascular Surgery. Nov 2012;**144**(5):1051-1060

[74] Kamata J, Kawazoe K, Izumoto H, et al. Predictors of sinus rhythm restoration after Cox maze procedure concomitant with other cardiac operations. The Annals of Thoracic Surgery. 1997;**64**(2):394-398

[75] Ad N, Holmes SD, Patel J, et al. The need for consistent predictors of success for surgical ablation of atrial fibrillation: A call to action. Innovations (Phila). 2017;**12**(6):421-429

[76] Gillinov AM, Sirak J, Blackstone EH, et al. The Cox maze procedure in mitral valve disease: Predictors of recurrent atrial fibrillation. The Journal of Thoracic and Cardiovascular Surgery. 2005;**130**:1653-1660

[77] Pecha S, Ghandili S, Hakmi S, et al. Predictors of long-term success

after concomitant surgical ablation for atrial fibrillation. Seminars in Thoracic and Cardiovascular Surgery. 2017;**29**(3):294-298

[78] Gelsomino S, La Meir M, Van Breugel HN, et al. Surgical ablation in patients undergoing mitral valve surgery: Impact of lesion set and surgical techniques on long-term success. Europace. 2015;**18**:1528-1537

[79] Loardi C, Alamanni F, Veglia F, et al. Modified Maze procedure for atrial fibrillation as an adjunct to elective cardiac surgery: Predictors of mid-term recurrence and echocardiographic follow-up. Texas Heart Institute Journal. 2015;**42**(4):341-347

[80] Ad N, Holmes SD, Stone LE, et al. Rhythm course over 5 years following surgical ablation for atrial fibrillation. European Journal of Cardio-Thoracic Surgery. 2015;**47**:52-58

[81] Gu W, Guo H, Lu C, et al. Surgical ablation for persistent atrial fibrillation in concomitant cardiac surgery: Mid-long-term result. European Journal of Cardio-Thoracic Surgery. 2017;**52**(5):888-894

[82] Jais P, Cauchemez B, Macle L, et al. Catheter ablation versus antiarrhythmic drugs for atrial fibrillation: The A4 study. Circulation. 2008;**118**:2498-2505

[83] DiBiase L, Mohanty P, Mohanty S, et al. Ablation versus Amiodarone for treatment of persistent atrial fibrillation in patients with congestive heart failure and an implanted device: Results from the AATAC Multicenter randomised trial. Circulation. 2016;**133**:1637-1644

[84] Virk SA, Bennett RG, Chow C, et al. Catheter ablation versus medical therapy for atrial fibrillation in patients with heart failure: A meta-analysis of randomised controlled trials. Heart, Lung & Circulation. 2019;**28**(5):707-718

[85] Packer DL, Mark DB, Robb RA, et al. Catheter ablation versus antiarrhythmic drug therapy for atrial fibrillation (CABANA) trial: Study rationale and design. American Heart Journal. 2018;**199**:192-199

[86] Phan K, Phan S, Thiagalingam A, et al. Thoracoscopic surgical ablation versus catheter ablation for atrial fibrillation. European Journal of Cardio-Thoracic Surgery. 2016;**49**(4):1044-1051

[87] Scanavacca M, Pisani CF, Hachul D, et al. Selective atrial vagal denervation guided by evoked vagal reflex to treat patients with paroxysmal atrial fibrillation. Circulation. 2006;**114**:876-885

[88] Di Biase L, Burkhardt JD, Mohanty P, et al. Left atrial appendage: An underrecognized trigger site of atrial fibrillation. Circulation. 2010;**122**:109-118

[89] Maesen B, Van-Loo I, Pison L, La-Meir M. Surgical ablation of atrial fibrillation: Is electrical isolation of the pulmonary veins a must? Journal of Atrial Fibrillation. 2016;**9**(1):1426

[90] Zeng Y, Cui Y, Li Y, Liu X, Xu C, Han J, et al. Recurrent atrial arrhythmia after minimally invasive pulmonary vein isolation for atrial fibrillation. The Annals of Thoracic Surgery. 2010;**90**(2):510-515

[91] On YK, Park KM, Jeong DS, et al. Electrophysiologic results after thoracoscopic ablation for chronic atrial fibrillation. Annals of Thoracic Surgery. 2015;**100**(5):1595-1602; discussion 1602-3

[92] Kron J, Kasirajan V, Wood MA, et al. Management of recurrent atrial arrhythmias after minimally invasive surgical pulmonary vein isolation and ganglionic plexi ablation for atrial fibrillation. Heart Rhythm. 2010;**7**(4):445-451

[93] Pison L, La Meir M, van Opstal J, et al. Hybrid thoracoscopic surgical and

transvenous catheter ablation of atrial fibrillation. Journal of the American College of Cardiology. 2012;**60**(1):54-61

[94] Gillinov M, Soltesz E. Surgical treatment of atrial fibrillation: Today's questions and answers. Seminars in Thoracic and Cardiovascular Surgery. 2013;**25**(3):197205

[95] Lee R, Vassallo P, Kruse J, et al. A randomized, prospective pilot comparison of 3 atrial appendage elimination techniques: Internal ligation, stapled excision, and surgical excision. The Journal of Thoracic and Cardiovascular Surgery. 2016;**152**(4):1075-1080

[96] Reddy VY, Sievert H, Halperin J, et al. Percutaneous left atrial appendage closure vs warfarin for atrial fibrillation: A randomized clinical trial. Journal of the American Medical Association. 2014;**312**(19):1988-1998

[97] Holmes DR Jr, Doshi SK, Kar S, et al. Left atrial appendage closure as an alternative to warfarin for stroke prevention in atrial fibrillation: A patient-level meta-analysis. Journal of the American College of Cardiology. 2015;**65**(24):2614-2623

[98] Friedman DJ, Piccini JP, Wang T, et al. Association between left atrial appendage occlusion and readmission for thromboembolism among patients with atrial fibrillation undergoing concomitant cardiac surgery. Journal of the American Medical Association. 2018;**319**(4):365-374

[99] Tsai YC, Phan K, Munkholm-Larsen S, et al. Surgical left atrial appendage occlusion during cardiac surgery for patients with atrial fibrillation: A meta-analysis. European Journal of Cardio-Thoracic Surgery. 2015;**47**(5):847-854

[100] Ailawadi G, Gerdisch MW, Harvey RL, et al. Exclusion of the left atrial appendage with a novel device: Early results of a multicenter trial. The Journal of Thoracic and Cardiovascular Surgery. 2011;**142**(5):1002-1009

[101] Whitlock R, Healey J, Vincent J, et al. Rationale and design of the left atrial appendage occlusion study (LAAOS) III. Annals of Cardiothoracic Surgery. 2014;**3**:45-54

[102] Melduni RM, Schaff H, Lee HC, et al. Impact of left atrial appendage closure during cardiac surgery on the occurrence of early postoperative atrial fibrillation, stroke, and mortality: A propensity score-matched analysis of 10,633 patients. Circulation. 2017;**135**(4):366-378

[103] Emmert MY, Puippe G, Baumüller S, et al. Safe, effective and durable epicardial left atrial appendage clip occlusion in patients with atrial fibrillation undergoing cardiac surgery: First long-term results from a prospective device trial. European Journal of Cardio-Thoracic Surgery. 2014;**45**(1):126-131

[104] Caliskan E, Sahin A, Yilmaz M, et al. Epicardial left atrial appendage AtriClip occlusion. Reduces the incidence of stroke in patients with atrial fibrillation undergoing cardiac surgery. Europace. 1 Jul 2018;**20**(7):e105-e114

[105] Available from: www.atricure.com

[106] Robertson JO, Saint LL, Leidenfrost JE, Damiano RJ Jr. Illustrated techniques for performing the Cox-Maze IV procedure through a right minithoracotomy. Annals of Cardiothoracic Surgery. 2014;**3**:105-116

[107] Beaver TM, Hedna VS, Khanna AY, Miles WM, et al. Thoracoscopic ablation with appendage ligation versus medical therapy for stroke prevention: A proof of concept randomised trial. Innovations (Phila). 2016 Mar-Apr;**11**(2):99-105

[108] Available from: www.bostonscientific.com